THE PHYSICIAN AS TEACHER

THE PHYSICIAN AS TEACHER

THOMAS L. SCHWENK, M.D.

Associate Professor
Department of Family Practice
Assistant Professor
Department of Postgraduate Medicine
  and Health Professions Education
The University of Michigan Medical School
Ann Arbor, Michigan

NEAL A. WHITMAN, Ed.D.

Associate Professor and
  Director of Educational Development
Department of Family and Preventive Medicine
University of Utah School of Medicine
Salt Lake City, Utah

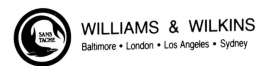

WILLIAMS & WILKINS
Baltimore • London • Los Angeles • Sydney

Editor: John N. Gardner
Associate Editor: Linda Napora
Copy Editor: Elia A. Flanegin
Design: Saturn Graphics
Illustration Planning: Wayne Hubbel
Production: Anne G. Seitz

Copyright © 1987
Williams & Wilkins
428 East Preston Street
Baltimore, MD 21202, U.S.A.

Printed in the United States of America

First Edition

Library of Congress Cataloging-in-Publication Data

Schwenk, Thomas L.
　The physician as teacher.

　Bibliography: p.
　Includes index.
　1. Medicine–Study and teaching.　2. Teacher-student relationships.　I. Whitman, Neal.　II. Title.
R834.S317　　1987　　　610.73'07'11　　　86-26716
ISBN 0-683-07613-2

Printed at the Waverly Press, Inc.

87 88 89 90 91　　　10 9 8 7 6 5 4 3 2 1

To my parents, Lee and Joanna,
who taught me to want to be happy, and
To my wife, Jane,
who taught me how.

T.L.S.

To my brother, Dr. Malcolm Whitman,
his wife, Elaine, and three daughters,
Meredith, Melissa, and Joanne.

N.A.W.

Foreword

I jumped at the chance to write the Foreword to this book - *The Physician as Teacher*. Grappling with the subject matter has been one of my obsessions for 30 years and whenever the topic is mentioned, I begin to articulate my thoughts with talk and pen. This, I am sure, is done to the consternation of those around me. I react, I suppose, to a request to discuss the importance of the doctor as a teacher like an old fireman who hears the alarm that beckons him to action.

I have always believed that doctoring and teaching have a lot in common. Patients cannot always make an independent judgment about the quality of patient care, but they can always determine how much physicians give of themselves. Medical students judge teachers just as patients judge physicians. Students judge the quality of teaching by determining how much teachers give of themselves.

Teaching and doctoring have a lot in common. Yesterday I had the following experience.

Mrs. Smith, a 78-year-old woman with severe obstructive pulmonary disease, was sitting in her hospital bed waiting for me to discuss the problems associated with a 6-cm aneurysm of the proximal portion of her aorta. The patient's two sons, her brother and his wife were also present. A medical student, medical resident, and Chief Medical Resident were with me.

Two teaching sessions transpired. The first one occurred inside the hospital room as I discussed my medical decision with the patient and her family. The second teaching session was with the student and residents. It, of course, took place a few minutes later, after we had left the patient's room. This is what happened.

Inside the patient's room I said, "Mrs. Smith, I have carefully considered your problem and I do not recommend surgical removal of the aneurysm."

The patient's son said, "What can we expect?" He had previously stated in front of his mother that they did not want to sit around until the aneurysm burst.

All aspects of the problem had been previously discussed with him and his mother and I had hoped he understood. It was, however, now clear that he did not understand.

So, I began again my effort to explain. As I spoke to him I cautioned myself to be patient. Feedback is essential for any teaching endeavor and I tried again. I responded, "You see, if she were younger, did not have severe lung disease, and the operative risk was 2–5%, it would be wise to have the surgeon remove the aneurysm and transplant the coronary arteries to the graft used to replace the aorta. But she is 78 years of age. She is active, happy, and has no pain. Her only symptom is hoarseness. The chance of rupture within 5 years is about 10–20% per year. The risk of surgery is 15–20% and the chance of a complication is high because there is a clot within the aneurysm. I believe there is a chance the clot may organize near the wall of the aneurysm and offer her some protection."

More was said in the room than I was accustomed to hearing in similar circumstances. Mrs. Smith, however, undoubtedly had such discussions prior to her referral to me. She did not seem disturbed by the discussion. I realized that to accomplish an acceptable therapeutic goal for Mrs. Smith it was necessary to ask the appropriate questions that would stimulate answers that would make it self-evident what should be done. So, I asked, "Mrs. Smith, what do you like to do?"

She answered something like this, "Keep my house, go for walks, and see my family."

I said, "Good. I think you should keep doing that."

The daughter-in-law asked, "Don't you think she should have an alarm system on her wrist that will signal the hospital?"

I gently responded, "I don't want her to live with that type of fear. I am hopeful she will not need such an alarm system. Remember, the goal is to let her live the happy life she has planned for herself."

I respectfully suggested that they seek another opinion because I did not claim that I knew all the answers. Mrs. Smith said no to that suggestion. She then took over the conversation by thanking me for the time and patience involved in concluding that we do nothing. She really was happy with the decision and indicated she would continue to do the things that made her happy.

The big question had been, "Mrs. Smith, what do you like to do?"

Later, with the student and residents, we discussed the conversation. They understood the deeper meaning of it all. They had previously looked up the scientific data on the chances the aneurysm might rupture in 5 years. They had talked with the surgeon about the operative risk of the procedure. They had studied the results of the pulmonary function test. They had considered all of the proper variables that had to be considered in order to arrive at a decision. Now was the time to think a little deeper about certain aspects of the problem. I asked, "Oh, by the way, what do you think about when you listen to the heart? I always found the three-step process to be useful. When we meet again tell me what you think about when you listen to the heart. For example, with Mrs. Smith it is possible to establish a differential diagnosis, based on auscultation alone, that includes aneurysm of the proximal portion of the aorta. Can you do that?"

The next day we discussed the matter again. After much discussion, we concluded that the three-step approach to auscultation of the heart was first to hear the sounds and murmurs, then to determine the altered pathophysiology that could cause the abnormal sounds (this implies that one knows the physiologic mechanisms of normal sounds), and then to create a differential diagnosis of the disease processes (etiology) that could cause the altered pathophysiology.

What do the two teaching sessions have in common? The session with the patient and her family and the sessions with the student and residents had the following in common: asking a question that required a thought process to take place in the listener; feedback from the listener to the teacher that indicated that communication and thinking took place; patience; the teacher indicated that he did not know everything; the giving of time to the patient and to the student and residents.

So, doctoring and teaching have much in common.

I have written on the nuances of this subject before. The following quotations are from *Notes From a Chairman* (Hurst JW: *Notes From a Chairman*. Chicago, Year Book Medical Publishers, 1987, pp 48–49) and are reproduced with permission from the publisher.

- Socrates taught by asking very simple questions. He did not say much but his questions made his student think. The trick is to play Socrates yourself and, at the same time, be Socrates' student. In other words, ask yourself questions—make yourself think.

- *Good* teaching can be identified when a teacher is able to start engines. *Excellent* teaching can be identified when a teacher is able to stimulate a student to start his or her own engine.

- The best way to judge students is by the quality of the questions they ask themselves. But we don't check that in an orderly fashion.

- Good doctors always prescribe a part of themselves (time and concern for their patients). Good teachers always give a part of themselves (time and concern) to their "students."

I again thank Drs. Schwenk and Whitman for asking me to write this Foreword. They have written an excellent book on an important subject. Physicians interested in teaching their patients or teaching their trainees should read, think, and practice the concepts of teaching that are set forth in this book.

J. Willis Hurst, M.D.
Candler Professor of Medicine (Cardiology)
Emory University School of Medicine
Chief of Cardiology
Emory University Hospital and Emory Clinic
Atlanta, Georgia

Preface

The purpose of this book is to help the physician become a better teacher. Why should a physician want to become a better teacher? First, there is a bit of historical tradition. The word "doctor," of course, derives from the Latin *docere*, which means "to teach." Long before physicians had tests to order, medications to prescribe, or surgeries to perform, their work was characterized by its educational value to patients and aspiring students.

The second reason a physician might want to become a better teacher is that physicians do a lot of teaching. Full-time academic physicians are the ones who most need to learn how to teach. We wrote this book primarily for them. The recent trend in academic medical centers is to hire physicians for their research skills—which will get them promoted—and their patient care skills—which will generate clinical revenue for the medical school and teaching hospital. Rarely, are academic physicians hired for their teaching skills, yet they are immediately given major, continuing teaching responsibilities with little or no attention to training. We offer this book to partially remedy this deficiency.

Another group of physicians has an almost equal need for improved teaching skills: practicing physicians. Why? Practicing physicians frequently hold clinical faculty positions and teach medical students and residents in their offices. They also are asked by hospitals with which they are affiliated to organize or make presentations to fellow medical staff members, nurses, administrators, and other health professionals. Physicians who act as civic leaders have teaching responsibilities in local community, political, and religious groups. In addition, every physician-patient encounter, perhaps several thousand in a year, may include some bit of teaching. The principles and techniques in this book are applicable to all of these situations.

The third and final reason physicians might want to improve their teaching skills is embodied in the well-known phrase, "to teach is to learn twice" (Joubert, as quoted in Raimi) and the Whitman-Schwenk corollary, "to teach well is to learn twice as well." There is ample evidence that in any teacher-learner encounter, the teacher learns more than the learner—one of the paradoxes of life, perhaps, but true nonetheless. Medical practice is enhanced, and its excellence furthered, by taking responsibility for medical teaching. When the student questions why the academic internist prescribed a certain medication, when the chief surgical resident questions the practicing surgeon's surgical technique, when the hospital nursing staff asks the local family physician to lecture on a favorite topic—in all situations—the physician-teacher inevitably learns more than the learners, and the quality of patient care is enhanced.

For these three reasons, and because of the pride we all have in offering to others our hard-won wisdom and experience, we are certain of the physician's need for improving his or her teaching skills, and almost as certain of the value of this book in satisfying part of that need. We each have yet to do our best teaching, and we hope physicians pursue excellence in their teaching as enthusiastically and thoroughly as they do in their practice of medicine.

Contents

PART ONE

Teaching as a Form of Communication

Part One presents the book's basic model, that teaching is a form of communication. These chapters address several types of communication that are relevant to teaching. The authors' aim is to encourage physicians to use and practice communication skills that they already possess in order to improve their teaching.

CHAPTER 1

Physicians as Communicators

It is curious that so many of our most important responsibilities are undertaken without significant preparation. Marriage and parenthood are probably the most ubiquitous illustrations, and there is little reason to expect that these states will ever evolve rationally. The task of medical teaching, on the other hand, is accepted deliberately and dispassionately, yet the preparation for that influential role is equally frail (Miller 1980).

Many efforts by physicians to pursue some type of instruction on teaching, such as reading a book on teaching skills or attending a workshop on faculty development, meet with less than astounding success. (After all, if the reader were already a master teacher, why would he[a] be reading this book?) Why are so many well-intentioned efforts at developing the teaching skills of physicians so modestly successful? One major reason is that medical teaching has been taught in the same manner as other disciplines in medicine: students are taught an isolated field of study with specialized concepts and

---

[a] It should be noted at this point that our readers are both male and female, of course, but our text consistently uses the pronoun *he* (or *his*). Although the he/she construction may reduce gender bias, we feel that it makes awkward reading. Our intention is not to promote sex stereotyping, but simply to provide concise writing.

jargon. Similarly, physicians wishing to improve their teaching skills are confronted with a profusion of rules and paradigms that bear little relationship to their past experiences. These ideas are usually presented in a language that is as foreign as Latin is to most physicians. Physician teachers are asked to adopt skills that do not apply to their immediate needs and to accept principles that are too theoretical for the realities of a physician's usually hectic life. In summary, physician teachers who have either excellent or dismal teaching skills acquired these skills intuitively regardless of any formal teacher training they may have received.

So how might this apparent gap between the training and performance of physician teachers be bridged? One way, which is also the basic premise of this book, is to approach learning as a basic human experience, and teaching as a basic interpersonal communication skill that is intuitive to physicians. Physicians possess powerful communication abilities that are derived from providing patient care. Given a chance, physicians have the natural ability to become excellent teachers. Thus instead of forcing more theoretical principles into the reader's already brimming store of medical and scientific facts, this book seeks to build upon the strong sense of communication that is inherent in the physician's interpersonal repertoire. Darley and Turner wrote in 1950 that "it is logical . . . that medical faculties are distrustful of principles that have been arrived at by teaching young children or by studying rats and other laboratory animals." Since this skepticism is still well placed in 1986, this book will not risk creating further skepticism by presenting impractical theories.

We believe that teaching is an interpersonal communicative event that occurs because of the physician's concern and desire to help. The same concern that a physician teacher has for his patient is revealed in his concern for his student as an individual. Similarly, the physician teacher's desire to help his patient translates into helping his student gain new knowledge, attitudes, and skills that will help the learner become a competent physician and future colleague. Holcomb and Garner (1973, p. vii) have noted, when describing excellent medical teachers, that "the reasons for their excellence in teaching are many, but perhaps the single most important reason for their teaching success is their sincere and deep interest in helping students learn." More specifically, as noted in a bulletin from the University of Michigan Center for Research on Learning and Teaching (Ericksen & Riskind 1971, p. 6), "what is important then is not to accept any one style of teaching as ideal but rather to recognize that 'good teaching' is defined in part by how well a teacher understands and communicates with his students."

If the reader is willing to accept, at least partially, the notions that (1) teaching is best studied not as a formal intellectual discipline, but rather as a type of normal interpersonal communication, and (2) physicians already possess considerable related communication experience, then brief examination of some other communication relationships might offer some guidelines and help. Some essential communication features of everyday relationships that physicians might already engage in, such as the employer-employee, parent-child, and physician-patient relationships, are directly applicable to medical teaching skills. Specifically, behaviors from these relationships apply directly to the critical components or objectives of effective medical teaching outlined by Skeff and associates (1984):

1. Communication of goals—the processes by which the teacher reveals his expectations of the learners.
2. Feedback and evaluation—the ways by which the teacher provides helpful information, or final evaluations, on the learners' performance and abilities.
3. Learning climate—the tone and educational ambience of the teaching setting that determines whether learners are stimulated or bored, and whether they can comfortably participate in a genuine way that reveals their strengths and weaknesses.
4. Control of the teaching session—the process by which the teacher keeps the session paced and focused so that it meets the needs of the teacher and the learner.

5. Increased understanding and retention—the techniques by which a teacher enhances the learners' understanding and retention of the discussion by stating the basis for the teacher's ideas and opinions, permitting questions to check understanding, emphasizing the relevance of the information to the learner (and ultimately a patient), and repeating and summarizing in relevant terms.
6. Stimulation of continued self-learning—the processes by which a teacher encourages learners to voluntarily continue learning beyond the goals or time set for a particular course.

The Employer-Employee Relationship

Of the considerable literature on constructive characteristics of employer-employee communication, Blanchard and Johnson's (1982) *The One-Minute Manager* is particularly adaptable to teaching. Interestingly, the second author of this book is a physician trained at the Harvard Medical School and the Mayo Clinic and Foundation. This small but invaluable book begins with a description of effective managers as those who "manage themselves and the people they work with so that both the organization and the people profit from their presence." Similarly, effective teachers are those whose method of teaching benefits the teacher, the learner, the teaching setting (e.g., hospital ward or medical office), and the learner's future patients. The *One-Minute Manager* offers three "secrets" of effective management that are equally applicable to effective teaching. These are presented next.

Clarifying the Learning Objectives

The *first secret* proposes that employers should help employees understand exactly what their responsibilities are and exactly what performance standards are necessary to meet those responsibilities.

This proposal by Blanchard and Johnson is directly applicable to Skeff's (1984) objective that the physician teacher clearly communicate the goals of teaching and learning. For example, at the start of a clerkship, preceptorship, or rotation, the physician teacher must tell the student or resident specifically what the learning objectives are and what specific activities will help the learner meet those objectives. This may require considerable discussion and negotiation with the student and may be done more implicitly for residents who are rotating as part of a residency program with specific overall objectives, but it must be done nonetheless.

Communicating Positive Feedback

The *second secret* advises employers to make sure, "in no uncertain terms," that the employee understands when he or she is doing something well. As Blanchard and Johnson (1982) put it, "Catch them doing something right." Most physicians are fairly good at giving positive feedback to learners at later times, however, the correct time to give it is immediately after a learner has performed well. Positive feedback is relatively easy to give in the presence of the patient, other health care personnel, or students. Waiting until some more formal time for delivering positive feedback (such as the end of the day, the end of the rotation, or the regularly scheduled advisor meeting 2 months hence) unfortunately delays the "good news" and dilutes their impact.

Communicating Negative Feedback

The *third secret* tells employers to ensure that the employee understands when he or she is doing something *wrong*. Not only do physician teachers infrequently criticize learners but they rarely do it at the time the learner performs poorly. Physicians generally do not want to be "bad guys (or gals)" and are usually uncomfortable giving negative feedback. Unsurprisingly, 4 to 8 weeks after the unmentioned error has occurred the student or resident is shocked at receiving a bad evaluation, and rightly so. Physician teachers must remember that medical teaching is a huge responsibility and that well-placed (i.e., shortly after the incorrect behavior) negative feedback is a critical part of that responsibility. Blanchard and Johnson (1982) also note that the "one-minute reprimand" should be followed by a reaffirmation of the employee's (i.e., student's) personal worth and general value to the organization. (This concept is discussed in greater detail in chapter 4.)

The second and third "secrets" of good employee management are directly applicable to Skeff's (1984) objective of giving students and residents information about their current clinical or academic performance so that they can either improve poor performance or continue to perform well.

The Parent-Child Relationship

From the wealth of excellent research on the communication characteristics of the parent-child relationship, some of the most useful work is found in *Parent Effectiveness Training* [(PET) Gordon 1970]. Interestingly, these principles also have been applied to teaching at the secondary school level in *Teacher Effectiveness Training* (Gordon 1975), and certain aspects apply equally well to medical teaching. PET describes an approach for parents working with children (theirs and others) based on intense active listening, so as to understand at both a factual and emotional level what children are saying. This is, of course, quite similar to active listening taught in basic patient interviewing courses. PET describes a method with which to constructively address children during a confrontation and to negotiate a "win-win" solution satisfactory for both parent and child. As part of this style of communication, 12 types of parental communications are described in the book, along with their potential for positive and negative effects on children. These 12 styles have directly analogous behaviors in teachers, and the effects on medical students and residents are also quite similar. This direct applicability does not imply that medical education is like secondary school teaching but rather that PET takes a particularly adult approach to teaching students of all ages.

Styles of Parental Communication

These 12 behaviors or styles (Gordon 1970) are directly useful in accomplishing Skeff's (1984) objectives of setting a helpful learning climate and controlling the tone and pace of the teaching-learning relationship:

Ordering, directing, commanding. While sometimes necessary, these behaviors often result in humiliated and/or rebellious students. Publically yelling at a medical student is demeaning and almost never justified, except perhaps in medical crises.

Warning, admonishing, threatening. Although the demonstration of power here is more subtle than in the first style above, the adverse effects on learners are the same.

Moralizing, preaching, obliging. Using moral ethical or professional failure to stimulate guilt has the effect of developing covert or passive resistance in the learner. Teachers may sometimes try to use arguments in favor of a certain test or treatment approach that are based more on personal bias than on scientific evidence. This type of influence will be short-term at best, and the teacher's credibility and opportunity to exert a long-term influence on students will dwindle.

Advising, giving suggestions or solutions. This style approaches the collegial relationship that is most effective in medical teaching. However, frequent advice giving may imply that the learner is inferior to the teacher, and the teacher may end up caring more about the particular patient problem or situation than does the learner. This is particularly important with senior residents who (presumably) are at a level of experience where more support and confirmation of medical skills is needed rather than advice on how to "do it best." A more supportive approach by the teacher encourages the senior resident to ask for help from the teacher and to view the instructor as a mentor rather than as a busybody.

Persuading logically, arguing, instructing, lecturing. This is the usual medical teaching style of the "teacher as expert," but good teaching requires more than just dispensing scientifically based facts. A teacher who bases most of his interactions with students on intellectual weight denies the interpersonal nature of the teacher-learner relationship that requires the teacher to understand the student as a person with needs that are not always rational.

Judging, criticizing, disagreeing, blaming. Feedback and evaluation are essential, but attacks on self-esteem and self-worth are not. Comments such as the one about the surgical resident "not being fit to be a butcher" are not only demeaning, they are unhelpful criticisms because they do not offer the learner any insight as to his specific professional deficiency. In addition, the surgical resident has a hard time accepting later feedback from this surgeon-teacher.

Praising, agreeing, evaluating positively, approving. Accurate and well-timed approval is helpful, but excessive or gratuitous approval can be condescending and insulting. The attending who tells all students their workups are excellent and show "evidence of great promise and hard work" will ultimately lack credibility as much as the charlatan or the abusive teacher.

Name-calling, ridiculing, shaming. These devastating attacks on a learner's self-esteem have absolutely no place in teaching (or in any other interpersonal relationship, for that matter).

Interpreting, analyzing, diagnosing. A rigorous and thorough analysis in which the learner participates *actively* is a powerful teaching tool. The chief resident who masterfully interprets a set of blood gases from a complex pulmonary patient without *fully* involving the third-year clerks has advanced his own learning, not theirs.

Reassuring, sympathizing, consoling, supporting. When genuine, this behavior is critical; unfortunately it is rarely expressed. Reassurance and support are almost impossible to overdo, but most medical teachers seem to subscribe to the theory that "If I could make it through this horrible, stressful process, so can they!"

Probing, questioning, interrogating. Questioning is the core behavior in medical teaching, but manipulation and the resulting learner resentment is a risk. Many teachers seem not to advance beyond the guess-what-I'm-thinking style of questioning: "I can think of only one reasonable cause of this patient's abdominal pain. What is it?" This type of teacher is usually remembered more for his malignancy than for his contributions as a medical educator.

Withdrawing, distracting, humoring, diverting. These can be important adjuncts to teaching, but, when used inappropriately or excessively, can trivialize the "teachable moment".

None of these behaviors is always "good" or always "bad" for the teacher-learner relationship (except for name-calling or ridiculing, which is _always_ bad), but using several of these behaviors discreetly and flexibly enhances the physician's teaching style. One's basic style of interpersonal communication is not limited to just a few behaviors, so why should one's teaching style be so limited?

The Physician-Patient Relationship

The third relationship, with which the physician is probably most familiar and, presumably, most experienced, is the physician-patient relationship. Many disciplines including psychiatry, psychology, medicine, ethics, and communications have written about the physician-patient relationship. Chapter 3 describes specific communication skills with patients that have direct counterparts with learners. This chapter examines the relationship itself to discover characteristics that bear on the teacher-learner relationship.

Physicians already appreciate the tremendous power of the physician-patient relationship. An outstanding review by Dodge (1983) describes the influence of this relationship on patient satisfaction, knowledge, compliance, and outcomes. Patients feel that the most important characteristics of a physician that lead to high patient satisfaction are "knowledge, understanding, interest, sympathy, and encouragement" (Reader et al. 1957). These equally worthy qualities of an excellent teacher lead to high learner satisfaction. Patient compliance is markedly improved when the physician demonstrates a warm, sensitive, and compassionate manner that stimulates patient confidence. The same is true for the teacher's demeanor and the learner's willingness to work. Finally, patient outcomes are directly influenced by the physician's communication style. For example, the length of the postoperative hospital stay and amount of analgesia prescribed is strongly affected by the anesthesiologist's interpersonal behaviors (Egbert et al. 1964). Similarly, learning outcomes, such as learner behavior change or information retention, are strongly and positively influenced by the teacher who is knowledgeable, concerned, open, and enthusiastic. As already stated, being a knowledgeable expert is not enough in either the physician or teacher roles.

Dodge (1983) characterizes the physician-patient relationship as three important exchanges between two individuals:

1. An *exchange of information,* in which the patient provides subjective and objective information on illness and the physician gives a diagnosis and treatment;
2. An *exchange of emotion,* in which the patient and physician exchange feelings about themselves, and the illness;
3. An *exchange of meaning,* in which the patient communicates to the physician the patient's previous attempts to understand the illness and the physician offers a revised interpretation that the patient can accept.

These three exchanges have direct applications to the teacher-learner relationship, including Skeff's (1984) stress on the importance of providing feedback and evaluation, the use of techniques to increase understanding and retention of factual material, and the stimulation of further self-directed learning.

Exchange of Information

An effective exchange of information requires powerful listening, observational, and responding skills. Listening skills include demonstrating respect and concern for the student or resident by questioning, focusing, facilitating, paraphrasing, and being silent. All these behaviors serve to elicit accurate and important information from the learner; a lot of instruction will be worthless or redundant if the teacher does not assess what the student already knows.

Observational skills include looking for both verbal and nonverbal cues, such as patterns of speech and word choice, as well as skin color, facial expressions, gestures, and body posture. Any teacher who has confronted an auditorium full of medical students, half of whom are asleep and the rest slouched in their seats, will attest to the value of observing carefully for learner cues and adjusting the teaching accordingly.

Responding skills include verbal behaviors (Ley et al. 1976) such as giving important information first, avoiding jargon, using clear organization and specific instructions, and giving the student some choices in the courses of action that might be taken next. During a discussion on teaching rounds about a patient with chest pain, the teacher might give specific instructions about the need for cardiac isoenzyme testing, but might also give the resident a choice on using oral or transdermal nitrate therapy. The resident is then much more involved in the direct care of the patient and more focused on the potential learning.

Exchange of Emotion

In the exchange of emotion, the physician must demonstrate certain qualities in order for the physician-patient relationship to move from the initial stage of no commitment to a stage of confidence, and hopefully on to a stage of total commitment in which the relationship is stable. The teacher-learner relationship, while perhaps not as intense as the physician-patient relationship, progresses similarly. The teacher qualities that encourage this progression are the same:

1. Empathy—understanding the learner's emotional state;
2. Respect—accepting both the positive and negative qualities of the learner ["unconditional positive regard" (Rogers 1951)];
3. Warmth—expressing care, concern, and compassion for the learner's stresses and the difficult nature of medical education;
4. Concreteness—clarity and brevity in the formulation and understanding of the learner's needs and problems and the teacher's recommendations;
5. Genuineness—congruence between what the teacher says and how it is said (the teacher who expresses interest in the student's presentation while dictating a letter and answering a telephone call does not fool the student);
6. Self-disclosure—the willingness of the teacher to share personal feelings and experiences (perhaps the *most* powerful role-modeling behavior a teacher can have);
7. Commitment—the willingness by the teacher to deal with unpleasant matters or to confront the learner about inadequacies or problem behaviors.

Exchange of Meaning

In the exchange of meaning, teachers and learners approach their relationships with often markedly divergent past experiences and current expectations, which can result in conflict. This conflict must be resolved before any good can come from the interaction. This resolution requires skills in negotiation, which are described in chapter 4.

Summary

Certain characteristics of the employer-employee, parent-child, and physician-patient relationships have considerable applicability to the teacher-learner relationship. Of these three relationships, some physicians may not have experienced the first two, but certainly all physicians have experienced the third. Physician skills in communicating with patients have considerable utility in teaching. The next chapter will examine the characteristics of the teacher-learner relationship, in preparation for directly comparing skills as a physician communicator with those needed to be an effective teacher communicator.

CHAPTER 2

The Roles of Teachers and Learners

The teaching-learning process is a human transaction involving the teacher, learner, and learning group in a set of dynamic interrelationships. Teaching is a human relational problem. (Bradford 1958, p. 135)

The first chapter made two basic points. First, teaching is best studied as a type of normal interpersonal communication between two people, a teacher and a learner. Second, the considerable experience that physicians have with certain other interpersonal relationships has applicability to the physician's role as a teacher. This chapter examines more closely the roles of the teacher and learner and the conditions that facilitate communication between the two. As a "relational problem," successful teaching and learning requires that the teacher understand and make constructive use of four factors:

1. The role of the teacher and the knowledge, attitudes, and skills that the teacher brings to the relationship;
2. The role of the learner and the experiences and knowledge that the learner brings to the relationship;

3. The conditions or external influences that enhance the teaching-learning process;
4. The types of interactions themselves.

This chapter will address the first three factors; chapter 4 discusses the fourth.

The Role of the Teacher

Many physicians think that their only role as teacher is to be a reservoir of knowledge with information flowing randomly toward students. Unfortunately, as noted often by McKeachie (1969), expertise is not enough for good teaching. The physician's success in teaching will depend largely on his believing "that the teaching-learning process is basically a delicate human transaction, requiring skill and sensitivity in human relations" (Bradford 1958, p. 138). Knowledge is necessary but not a sufficient, in mathematical parlance, "quantity" to guarantee good teaching.

Beyond presenting information—after all, most medical facts can be found in journals and textbooks—the desire of most medical teachers is to make the practice of medicine understandable and meaningful. What the teacher can provide that does not appear in print is what one scientist called the "inner relevance" of the material (Kestin 1970). Clinicians do this when they personalize the material, relating their own patient-care experiences.

For example, an unattributed story describes the introductory lecture to sophomore medical students in the obstetrics/gynecology section of the organ systems course. The course director's goal was to get the students excited about the course. In addition, he wanted the students to anticipate with great interest and excitement their junior-year ob/gyn rotation. To achieve these goals, he presented a case in which doing the right thing at the right time made all the difference in the world. He presented a case of a pregnant woman carrying twins with twin transfusion syndrome in which one fetus transfuses blood to the other through a single placenta. Digoxin was given orally to the mother, resolving heart failure in the hemodynamically overloaded twin. After discussing the case, he introduced the mother and the twin boys to the class as the students rose in applause. In his introductory session, this course director was aiming at something other than a transfer of information; the remaining sessions would provide ample time for that. His purpose was to motivate students and to share his love for his chosen specialty. While this amount of drama may not be appropriate in every teaching session, this example clearly demonstrates that _how_ facts are presented is as important as _what_ is presented.

If the teacher, then, is not just a fountain of knowledge, what is he? Mann and his colleagues (1970) describe six roles that a teacher may assume to varying degrees. The degree to which each of these roles is adopted will characterize the physician's "style" as a teacher. Style is probably not as important as character or expertise, but may be a reflection of both.

Expert

The teacher is the source of all knowledge (the "reservoir of facts" described above) and there is considerable discrepancy between the teacher's level of experience and wisdom and that of the students. To close this gap is the reason for teacher and students to come together. The physician teacher may choose the role of expert in medical emergencies or while giving lectures in his area of expertise.

Formal Authority

The teacher is responsible to school administrators, specialty boards, and hospital credentials committees for evaluating and certifying student competency. The teacher upholds professional standards, and students depend on the teacher's evaluations. Residency directors, chiefs of service, department chairmen, and deans fulfill this role frequently.

Socializing Agent

The teacher is a member of a professional discipline and is accredited by a scholarly or professional society. Like the obstetrics/gynecology professor described earlier, the teacher embodies the values and attitudes of a profession which the student hopes to eventually join.

Ego Ideal

The teacher is a real-life example of a person whom students would someday like to become. The teacher is idealized by students in unimaginable ways. For example, every student remembers how impressed he was with the first physician whom he was allowed to observe practicing medicine. Chief residents, faculty advisors, ward attendings, and office preceptors have enormous role-modeling influences.

Facilitator

The teacher is aware of the needs and aspirations of students but does not automatically assume that he can provide everything the student needs. The teacher can listen, question, paraphrase, encourage, or disabuse students but cannot always act for them: "You can lead a horse to water", etc. Physician-teachers often assume the role of facilitator with senior residents or with graduate students in an advanced research seminar.

Person

The teacher and students feel sufficient mutual trust to share ideas, feelings, and thoughts. The teacher does not necessarily have to like the students but can accept their needs and imperfections. The teacher may provide significant personal help and support outside the formal teaching setting. This role may evolve over a long time, although not with every student. When the teacher and learner become close medical colleagues, the teaching-learning process has been successful.

The parallel is obvious between the roles and behaviors of a teacher and that of a physician providing patient care. There is a spectrum of physician behaviors, ranging from the physician as medical expert to the physician as person/friend, that is analogous to the spectrum of teaching roles defined by the six roles described above. Physicians may use part of these roles, to varying degrees, in any one teaching activity, but the usual mix defines the physician's style as a teacher. Most medical teachers are probably too much the expert and too little the mentor, facilitator, and friend. To the degree that physicians can move towards the latter direction, without forsaking the former, the resultant teaching style will be more successful.

The Role of the Learner

What do learners bring to the teacher-learner relationship? Bradford (1958) notes that learners are usually loaded with all sorts of anxieties, needs, problems, and "screens" that interfere with learning. How secure is the learner in the situation and group? "Does he perceive the teacher as capable of understanding and helping him? To what extent does he even recognize the kinds of help he would most appreciate as well as most need?" (Bradford 1958, p. 136). How motivated is the learner to learn and to risk giving up old ideas and knowledge for the sake of new ones? To what extent is self-esteem or self-image threatened by learning?

Mann et al. (1970) have described eight general types of students that are somewhat analogous to the six roles for teachers presented earlier. Of the eight, five types are most applicable to medical students and residents. (The other three types, *discouraged workers, heroes,* and *attention-seekers,* are rarely seen in medical settings.)

Compliant Students

These are the typical "good" learners who work hard, are task oriented, show little emotional turmoil, and are primarily concerned with understanding the material and complying with teacher requests.

Anxious-Dependent Students

This may be the predominant type in medical school; they are dependent on the teacher for knowledge and support and are anxious about evaluation. Feelings of anxiety and incompetence block these students from actively learning and make them more concerned about grades than actual learning. They are difficult to engage in discussion and prefer lectures.

Independent Students

These learners are often older than their counterparts and seem confident and unthreatened by the teacher. They favor peer relationships with the teacher and approach the material calmly, objectively, and often creatively. Medical students with previous graduate work and chief residents often fall into this category.

Sniper Students

These learners are uninvolved due to a low level of self-esteem and a high level of pessimism concerning their ability to form productive relationships with authority figures. They can be hostile, but are elusive when confronted with a particular issue. Every class has a few of these; they may go on to lackluster careers, always complaining and making excuses about mediocre efforts and performance.

Silent Students

These learners are characterized by what they do not do. They are notable for their lack of participation and the passivity of their learning, which may therefore be inadequate. They feel helpless and vulnerable, but without the anxiety characterizing the anxious-dependent learners.

Learners bring vastly different needs and agendas to their interactions with teachers just as patients do to their medical encounters. Teachers cannot be all things to all learners, just as physicians cannot provide medical care effectively for patients of all personality types. However, awareness of different types of learners and adjustment of the teacher's style insofar as is possible, will be helpful (chapter 4 will discuss how to adopt new teaching styles).

Conditions for Effective Learning

Medical students and residents are adult learners, and medical education should follow the principles of adult learning. Readers who do not find this statement absurd deserve applause. Many physicians, however, may disagree, if not consciously, at least in their manner of teaching. Despite the fact that medical learners are adults pursuing a difficult field of study requiring discipline and maturity, many of the basic assumptions underlying their current education would be recognizable to an elementary school teacher. How is this apparent paradox resolved and how can medical education become more of an adult learning process? The principles that enhance the teacher–adult learner relationship are discussed next.

Four Adult-Learning Principles

Adults prefer to apply what they learn shortly after learning it. This principle is violated frequently in basic science education, but perhaps less so in clinical teaching; it ought not to be violated at all. The challenge for teachers is to justify any teaching that cannot be shown to have some, albeit small or indirect, application to a relevant patient problem or clinical situation. Bedside teaching should focus on the findings and problems of the patient at hand. Lectures and grand rounds should include relevant case presentations. Other teaching should be case-based insofar as is possible.

Adults prefer learning concepts and principles rather than facts. This issue has, of course, been directly addressed in the Report of the Panel on the General Professional Education of the Physician (Association of American Medical Colleges 1984). Medical education suffers terribly under the weight of unrelated and sometimes relatively useless facts. As medical knowledge expands, so does the density of the medical education process, often to the detriment of the problem-solving and clinical-reasoning skills of future physicians. It is generally believed that the increasing rate of this information explosion precludes the learning of every new medical fact. This suggests that learning how to use facts is likely to be more helpful than accumulating additional facts, a task that is by definition impossible to do successfully in the long run. Therefore, teachers ought not to compound what is already recognized as a major problem by national authorities. To alleviate this problem, several medical schools (e.g., New Mexico, Southern Illinois, and Harvard) are pursuing major curricular redesigns that are case based and that emphasize clinical problem solving rather than fact learning (Barrows & Tamblyn 1980).

Adults like to help set their own learning objectives. "What!," the reader may ask. "How can students and residents possibly determine what they need to learn? Are they not 'unconsciously incompetent' (see chapter 8) by definition?" Yes and no. The teacher, of course, possesses considerable knowledge and experience that learners do not. However, just as the physician discusses or negotiates the objectives of a proposed treatment with a patient, the physician teacher should also negotiate with learners regarding appropriate educational objectives. These objectives, of course, may be limited by overall needs, resources, and goals. However, *all* instruction must include some previous assessment of experiences and negotiation of objectives. Assessment of objectives may be done directly, in the case of a resident in an office preceptorship, or more implicitly in the case of a new class of medical students. The teacher who does negotiate learning objectives will be pleasantly surprised at the remarkably positive effect this has on learner motivation.

Adults like to receive feedback to help them evaluate their own performance. Feedback for the sake of improving performance is called "formative evaluation." Formative evaluation is rarely offered compared with the numerous opportunities for making decisions about competence, promotion, or advancement (i.e., summative evaluation). Unfortunately, many physician teachers hesitate to make negative comments even though this might help a learner change professional behavior, make a better decision, or perform a skill more precisely. Well-intentioned formative evaluation is critical for cementing a teacher-learner relationship and successfully ending the learning process (chapter 4 further addresses these important skills).

Summary

In summary, the teacher-learner relationship is a communication relationship between two people, just like many other relationships of which the physician may be a part. The teacher has certain roles to play; these roles may vary according to the situation or learner, just as the physician varies his style with different patients in different situations. The learner has a role to play as well, and, like the patient, he tends to play the same role most of the time. These roles are played under certain conditions that strongly influence the relative success of the teacher-learner relationship. The next chapter examines some specific types of physician-patient interactions and shows how they are directly analogous to teacher-learner communications. Rather than require the reader to learn a whole new set of skills to become a better teacher, chapter 3 shows the physician-teacher how to adapt patient-care communication skills that are already familiar to him.

CHAPTER 3

The Teacher-Learner Relationship

A little boy tells his friend, "I taught Rover how to whistle!" With an ear up to the dog's face, the friend responds, "I don't hear him whistling." The first boy responds, "I said I taught him. I didn't say he learned it." (Anonymous)

Some teachers believe that if there was no learning there was no teaching. According to this view, the verb "to teach" is analogous to the verb "to give." When something is given, it is received. However, if something was never received, then it was never given. Proponents of this view recognize that an instructor may have tried to teach, but if there was no learning, then what the instructor did should not be called "teaching." The significance of this view is that a teacher may not be considered a good teacher just because he seemed to teach well. What counts is whether someone learned from that teacher (Machlup 1979).

Other teachers believe that teaching is *anything* done by an instructor that intentionally promotes learning. According to this view, the verb "to teach" is analogous to the verb "to offer." When something is offered, it may or may not be received. When something is taught, it may or may not be learned. Proponents of this view recognize that teaching may occur in circumstances so adverse that little learning may occur. The significance of this view is that the characteristics of good teaching can be identified (Donald & Shore 1977), despite the absence of learning. Both views have value. On one hand, teachers should be concerned with the outcome of their medical teaching: Did the residents or students learn? On the other hand, process is equally important: Did the teacher make a reasonable effort to do what is known to be effective? Teaching and learning comprise a two-way relationship, with both parties having responsibility for its success. This chapter will focus on this two-way relationship.

Teacher-Centered vs. Learner-Centered Instruction

The relationship between the teacher and residents or students is characterized by its "adultness." Because both the teachers and learners in medical education are adults, the term *andragogy* rather than *pedagogy* describes the art or profession of medical teaching. Pedagogy, like pediatrics, is concerned with children. Medical educators are concerned with adults. This distinction is often overlooked, or purposely denied in medical education, but its recognition can make an important difference in the teacher's outlook. The major principle of andragogy is that adults learn best when they are engaged as actively as possible in their own learning. Knox (1979), a pioneer in the field of adult education, commented that adults who wish to enhance their skills see themselves as "users" rather than as "recipients" of education. Similarly, McLagan (1978), another adult educator, emphasizes that when working with adults, the role of the teacher is to help learners develop knowledge, attitude, and skills, whereas, their actual development is the responsibility of the adult learner.

The notion that adults should be actively involved in their own learning and that the teacher's role is to facilitate the learning has led to an approach in instruction known as *learner-centered*. However, medical education is dominated by *teacher-centered* instruction. The teacher-centered approach holds that a topic must first be broken down into small units or stages, with each unit being divided into still smaller pieces of information. Through repetition and reinforcement, students learn the correct answers to questions about the small pieces of information. According to this approach, students progress through the units or stages until they learn the whole subject. Androgogical teachers call this approach "spoon feeding" and consider it somewhat condescending or gratuitous. Medical educators who believe in andragogy believe that the problem with medical education is that it is too teacher centered. Eichna (1980), who returned to medical school as a student for 4 years after retiring as the Chairman of the Department of Medicine at the State University of New York's Downstate Medical Center, also holds this view. As a student, he discovered that, "the emphasis is on the accumulation of facts. Fact is king." He observed that the emphasis on learning facts continued into the third and fourth years: "It is a mistake to hold that bedside teaching is necessarily equated to thinking and problem solving. Some undoubtedly is, but so much of it is minilecturing, noneducational chores, and the reflexive ordering of test after test."

Norman (1980), a psychology professor, has described how he began his teaching career with a teacher-centered view. At first he believed that all a teacher needed was a knowledge of the subject plus an understanding of what the students already knew, the teacher then simply filling in the differences between the two. Norman (1980, p. 39) started out with an appealing, but miscalculated, vision:

> Essentially, I had assumed that students were passive receptacles and that an ideal teaching situation would be one where the students would come into the classroom, unscrew the tops of their skulls, and the instructor could walk around the class, peer intently into the brain of each student and say something like, "Hmm, you seem to have this connection missing," and then proceed to add the necessary connections.

With experience, Norman found that his vision was not accurate. What the *students* did, rather than what he did, determined educational effectiveness. He discovered that students came to a learning situation with preexisting experiences and expectations. In their own ways, they tried to make sense of what was being taught. As described by Bradford (1958, p. 135), a cognitive scientist, "learning is not a matter of filling a void with information. It is a process of internal organization of a complex of thoughts, patterns, perceptions, assumptions, attitudes, feelings, and skills, and of successfully testing this reorganization."

Glassman (1980, p. 31), a medical school teacher of biochemistry and genetics, made a discovery about his teaching similar to Norman's:

> About five years ago, after years of moderate success as a university teacher of biochemistry and genetics, I made a discovery that has affected my teaching ever since. I was the one whose thinking skills were enhanced and whose creativity was stimulated. I played the active learning role; the students' role was passive, often consisting of listening and trying to decipher what I was trying to say during the lecture.

The implication for the medical educator is that the goal for students and residents is to move beyond learning new information to a higher order of learning, where learners answer their own questions and solve their own problems. As described by Knopke and Diekelman (1978), the student-centered approach in the health sciences means that lectures should be minimized and only used to teach essential information and that group discussions should be used to raise, discuss, and answer questions, with the teacher serving as a resource and guide.

Methods of Teaching

The principle that adults learn best when they are engaged as actively as possible in their own learning led Whitman (1981) to a model of teaching shown in Figure 3.1.

According to this model, there are basically only four universal methods of teaching. Two methods occur in the classroom:

1. A *lecture,* in which the teacher is active but the learner is passive;
2. A *group discussion,* in which a teacher and learner are both actively engaged.

Two methods occur in the "application" setting:

	Active teacher	Passive teacher
Active learner	Group discussion	Tutorial
Passive learner	Lecture Preceptorship	

Fig. 3.1 Active-passive model of teaching.

3. A *preceptorship*, in which the teacher is active but the learner is passive;
4. A *tutorial*, in which a learner is active and a teacher is passive.

An "application" setting refers to wherever learners use what they learned in the classroom. In medical education, it is known as "clinical education" and means wherever there are patients: hospitals, physician offices, nursing homes, or patient homes. Some medical educators use "preceptorship" to mean a rotation of a medical student or resident in a physician's office. However, "preceptorship" can be used in a more generic sense to mean any clinical experience in which the learner is relatively passive. In this sense, most clinical experiences for medical students are preceptorships. Medical students observe much but do little on their own. What they do is closely supervised and monitored. On the other hand, most clinical experiences for residents are tutorials in the sense that residents are relatively active. They do much on their own and often there is a lesser (although presumably an adequate) amount of supervision and monitoring.

According to a "learning vector" developed by Stritter and colleagues (1986), there should be a relationship between the amount of independence given to a medical student or resident and his level of maturity. Figure 3.2 shows that teachers should use instructional strategies that maintain dependence for learners with low maturity and promote independence for learners with high maturity. Figure 3.3 demonstrates the consequences of a mismatch—medical students or residents may feel anxiety when given too much independence and frustration when given too little. Anxiety or frustration in students or residents may be a cue to teachers that they are providing too much or too little independence in the clinical setting.

Active-Passive Models of Patient Care and Teaching

The relative degree of activity and passivity that the teacher and learner bring to their relationship greatly influences the specific be-

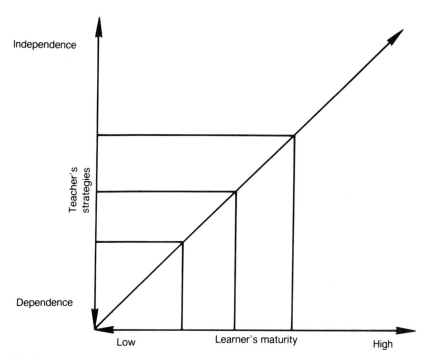

Fig. 3.2 Learning vector. [Adapted from Stritter et al. 1986.]

haviors or communication skills that are effective in the four basic methods of teaching. These communication skills and behaviors form the teacher's repertoire of teaching techniques upon which to draw. The specific communication skills appropriate to each of these methods are derived from, or have parallels in, the physician-patient relationship.

The physician-patient relationship has been well studied to determine the most effective and efficient communication behaviors. One model, which parallels the active-passive model for teachers and learners, describes the physician-patient relationship with two com-

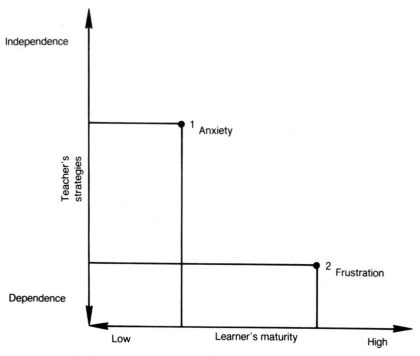

Fɪɢ. 3.3   Learning vector. [Adapted from Stritter et al. 1986.]

plementary control scales, along which physicians and patients move at equal rates and in the same directions.

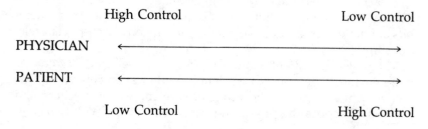

As the physician moves from left to right on the scale and uses interviewing and communication behaviors that are less and less assertive or controlling, the patient also moves from left to right and takes more control and responsibility for the relationship and its outcome. Both physician and patient could move from right to left on the control scale with opposite results: An extreme example of high physician control and low patient control would be when a physician interviews a patient who is mentally and legally incompetent. An example of an opposite situation to the far right of the scales would be a traditional psychoanalytic relationship in which the patient takes almost total responsibility for the outcome of the interaction and receives little feedback from the psychiatrist.

These scales, then, define physician and patient roles that are complementary in their levels of activity and passivity. In fact, these control designations can be replaced with active-passive designations, and the scales converted to a 2 × 2 matrix. This matrix (Fig. 3.4)

	Active physician	Passive physician
Active patient	2 Cooperative negotiation	1 Attentive silence
Passive patient	3 Persuasive confrontation	?

FIG. 3.4 Active-passive model of the physician-patient relationship.

is analogous to the active-passive model of teaching and learning. Three of the four boxes in Figure 3.4 are labeled according to the dominant characteristic of the relationship. The box in the lower right corner, in which both physician and patient are passive, is unlabeled; this "relationship", or lack of one, has yet to be defined.

The value of doing this tedious model building is that each of the three types of relationships defined between physician and patient has a repertoire of communication skills and behaviors applicable to both patient care and teaching.

Communication Skills in Clinical Care and Clinical Teaching

Attentive silence. Box 1 (Fig. 3.4) defines a relationship in which the patient is very active and the physician relatively passive. The patient is in control of pace, technique, and outcome. The communication skills used by the physician in this situation are

1. Attentive silence;
2. Observation;
3. Purposeful eye contact;
4. Tracking ("nods and grunts");
5. Open-ended encouragement and advocacy;
6. Surface paraphrasing.

These skills, as useful teaching techniques, will be described in the first part of chapter 4.

Cooperative negotiation. Box 2 (Fig. 3.4) contains a set of skills that define a relationship in which both physician and patient are active. One may take a more active role than the other at times, but the process is mutual, facilitative, and cooperative. Both physician and patient share responsibility for process and outcome of the interaction. Physician behaviors in this category include

7. Self-disclosure;
8. Active listening;
9. Intense paraphrasing;
10. Open-ended questioning;
11. Positive and negative feedback.

These communication skills and their corresponding teaching techniques are described more fully in the middle of chapter 4.
Persuasive confrontation. Box 3 (Fig. 3.4) defines skills in which the physician is active and the patient passive. Interviewing or communication skills in this category include

12. Summarizing;
13. Information and advice giving;
14. Critiquing and correcting;
15. Persuading.

With these behaviors or skills, the physician is clearly in control of the pace, the topic, the range of possible patient responses, and the outcome of the interview. The teaching skills that correspond to these interviewing skills will be discussed in detail at the end of chapter 4.

Summary

In summary, an active-passive model of the teacher-learner relationship shows that participants play complementary roles in the degree to which they take responsibility for the pace, technique, and outcome of the interaction. An analogous active-passive model of the physician-patient relationship describes the roles played by each participant, such that the specific interviewing and communication skills used by physicians with patients have teaching technique counterparts. The assertion that "teaching is like patient care, only more so" will be proven by describing these teaching techniques in chapter 4 as they derive directly from patient-care skills.

Attentive Silence, Negotiation and Challenge

The true teacher defends his pupils against his own personal experience (Alcott Bronson in Auden & Kronenberger, 1981).

In the ideal case, a contract is developed at the beginning of each teaching encounter. This need not be a long or complex process. Rather, a simple, brief exchange of thoughts about needs, expectations, roles, and content may take only one or two comments (Pratt and Magill, 1983).

The professor stepped up on the platform, and, by way of breaking the ice remarked, "I've just been asked to come up here and say something funny." At this point, a student heckler in the back of the hall called out, "You'll tell us when you say it, won't you?" The professor answered, "I'll tell *you*. The others will know!" (Braughman 1974, p. 124)

In chapter 3, we used a model based on the active-passive nature of the physician-patient relationship to identify three sets of communication skills applicable to teaching. These three sets of skills form a spectrum of 15 specific behaviors that can be applied to any teaching encounter of any format, although certainly not all will be used in any one encounter (Fig. 4.1). The three quotations might seem at first glance to be somewhat mutually exclusive depictions of the role of the teacher. Actually, they represent two anchor points and a middle ground on the spectrum of 15 behaviors and show that the repertoire

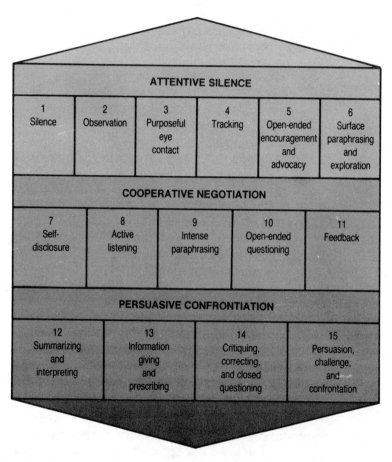

FIG. **4.1** Spectrum of 15 specific behaviors that can be applied to any teaching encounter.

of possible teaching behaviors is rich and nearly limitless. The job of the teacher is to pick the right set of behaviors to match the needs of the situation, the learning objectives, and, most importantly, the needs and style of the learner. This matching process will become clearer in chapters 5–9, which describe specific teaching formats common to medical education. In this chapter, the specific behaviors will be described, with examples showing how they apply in common medical teaching situations. We will start the discussion at the end of the spectrum representing the most passive form of physician-teacher behavior.

Attentive Silence

When the physician gives the patient control in an interview there is a set of facilitative skills labeled "attentive silence." These skills, which are helpful in eliciting a rich and accurate patient history, are also very important in teaching for a similar reason. Teachers are far more effective when they know what the learners know and do not know, what their attitudes and values are, and what learners can and cannot do. This assessment of learner needs makes it possible to target instruction accurately and allows teachers to meet the individual needs of students and residents (Whitman & Schwenk 1984). In fact, instruction is fundamentally impossible without an accurate picture of what the learner needs to learn, just as it is impossible to care for patients without knowing what they need and want. Unfortunately, physician teachers sometimes break this fundamental rule with both constituencies, although in our experience it occurs far more frequently with learners than with patients.

Assessment is easier when learners tell the teacher what their needs are. This is done, both directly and indirectly, when learners talk and teachers listen. Obviously this does not always happen. For example, a study by Foley et al. (1979) of teaching rounds in internal medicine showed that teachers were talking nearly two-thirds of the possible time and residents nearly one-third. Students "occupied the air waves" only 4% of the available time.

Given that teachers should talk less, there is still a concern about the accuracy of what they hear. Can teachers rely on what they hear from learners to help plan instruction, within the boundaries of the learning objectives that teachers have already set? For instance, in group discussions (discussed in chapter 6), medical students and residents are often expert at playing the "pretend to know" game in order to hide their ignorance. In one-on-one clinical teaching, how can teachers discourage learners from putting up a facade? One way is by establishing an open relationship with their learners so as to encourage helpful self-assessment and self-disclosure. Rogers (1951) has identified three conditions that are necessary in counselor-client relationships to encourage self-disclosure and trust. These conditions are equally applicable to the physician-patient and teacher-learner relationship and are particularly embodied in the skills of attentive silence.

First, teachers have to be *empathic,* i.e., they must perceive and understand another person's inner world. Second, teachers must be *congruent,* i.e., their words and actions have to accurately reflect true feelings and attitudes. Finally, teachers should show *positive regard* for the other person. In a study of elementary and high schools, Aspy and Roebuck (1977) demonstrated that teachers' levels of empathy, congruence, and positive regard are positively and significantly related to students' cognitive growth. Although this study has not been replicated in medical education, other related work reveals that learning is enhanced when physician teachers provide high levels of empathic understanding and unconditional positive regard. Attentive silence is critical, since there is no better way to demonstrate respect for a learner or to allow a learner to express himself clearly than for the teacher to be silent while the learner expresses himself.

The skills of attentive silence allow the teacher to communicate that he understands and accepts what the student is saying and that the student is free to continue his statement. This does not necessarily imply that everything the learner says is correct, just that it is helpful for both if the learner continues expressing himself a bit longer (Hansen et al. 1972). Skills of attentive silence range from absolute silence to superficial paraphrasing.

1. Silence

By remaining absolutely silent when the learner pauses, a teacher communicates that he understands what the learner has said. The silence provides the student or resident time to think and to continue to talk. Silence could, of course, suggest that the teacher is not listening, is asleep, or is thinking about his son's upcoming basketball game or a recent meeting with the department chairman. The teacher must indicate attentiveness through nonverbal behavior, such as facing the learner, maintaining intermittent eye contact, nodding (as opposed to dozing), or taking notes (as opposed to working on unrelated paperwork). For example, when a resident is presenting a patient for discussion and pauses at the end of the history, the teacher might show general support for the presentation to that point by nodding silently. When a student is performing a skin biopsy for the first time, using local anesthetic on an awake patient, the teacher can show silent approval to start suturing with a smile and a blink of the eyes if the student happens to look up at him.

2. Observation

In a certain sense, all interpersonal interactions in teaching come under the heading of "observation" (Mangold & Zaki 1982). In a teaching situation, the teacher is almost always observing the learner. However, as physicians know from practicing medicine, systematic observation of what the patient says or does not say and how it is said or not said offers valuable information to the physician. A teacher's observation of learners offers similar nonverbal cues, e.g., anxiety, depression, hesitancy, confidence, enthusiasm, boredom, resistance, sadness, discomfort, fear, or relief. Nonverbal messages frequently differ from verbal statements; the degree of congruence or discrepancy between the two can give further clues about the learner's emotional and cognitive states (Dittman 1963). A student's confused or blank look as he hesitantly sorts through surgical instruments on a tray and delays selecting one belies his confident assertion, "I've done lots of these biopsies!" A resident's sparkling eyes and light step as he turns to walk away may be the only acknowledgment a teacher gets for having praised the resident for a well-run cardiopulmonary resuscitation. Observing these behaviors and nonverbal cues may be all that is required to plan future teaching. The observations need not always be communicated directly to the learner, but this may be appropriate at times.

3. Purposeful Eye Contact

The teacher who uses purposeful eye contact is still silent and attentive but is purposefully staring at the learner. The teacher may want to indicate receptivity to what the learner is saying, suspicion or concern about what was just said, or encouragement if the learner wishes to reveal something important. This technique has infrequent use and may make some learners uncomfortable and less willing to volunteer feelings or thoughts. It has particular value with learners who are otherwise hard to engage, who seem to be avoiding the teacher, or who seem hesitant to present particular information or opinions and need to know that the teacher is particularly receptive. This might occur during the presentation of sensitive patient psychosocial information or the discussion of a patient's impending death.

4. Tracking

Sometimes it is helpful to use noncommittal words, or nonverbal messages such as "nods and grunts," to convey interest and keep the person talking. This is particularly true when the learner is somewhat less experienced and seems hesitant but is presenting or performing well and needs small amounts of encouragement. By saying, "I see," "OK," "Uh-huh," or "good," the teacher can communicate that he understands, or approves of, what the learner is saying or doing without interrupting the learner's momentum. This is helpful when time is short and the presentation needs to move along quickly, when the teacher is observing a correctly done psychomotor skill or procedure, or when a student is responding well to a direct question in a small group discussion.

5. Open-Ended Encouragement and Advocacy

General supportive statements build rapport, create a reservoir of goodwill, and encourage the learner to work harder and learn more. Much of medical education seems based on the notion that support and friendly helpfulness only create lazy, uncommitted medical students and residents. The principles of adult education suggest, however, that adult learners may learn best in a supportive, less-threatening environment. One of the critical principles of adult education described in research by Knox (1970) is the establishment of a low-anxiety, nonthreatening environment in which there is a strong and positive teacher-learner relationship. However, more recent research suggests that moderate levels of "facilitative" stress are actually most productive. "Facilitative" means that the teacher is well-intentioned and that the anxiety generated is the constructive anxiety of learning, rather than the fear of being made to feel stupid or personally demeaned. Making fun of students who mispronounce medical terminology, telling surgical residents they "are not fit to be butchers," or showing inappropriate and undue impatience with a student struggling to put on surgical gloves for the first time are not likely to build a strong and positive relationship. Here are some better examples:

Reflection.   Simply restating or reflecting a learner's thought or expressed feeling shows understanding and encouragement. Reflection does not necessarily imply approval, nor should a teacher suggest he completely understands what the student may be thinking or feeling. Because it might be more precise than the learner's own words, a teacher's restatement can be illuminating. However, restatement or reflection is not intended to push the learner into a particular position or to suggest a line of thought. For example, as a resident finishes presenting a complicated case and tentatively suggests cholecystitis as the diagnosis, the teacher can say, "So you think she has cholecystitis?," even if it seems quite clear that irritable bowel syndrome is the correct diagnosis. Reflection suggests that at least the learner's hard work and general thinking process are laudable, even if his answer is incorrect. When a student makes an obvious flippant remark that indicates considerable frustration, the teacher can say, "You seem a bit frustrated in caring for this patient," indicating that the frustration may be understandable but that the method of expression may not be. This mild rebuke is so gentle that the learner feels support rather than disapproval from the teacher.

Public demonstrations.   Nothing shows a learner that he is "part of the team" better than being included in discussions, decisions, and conversations. The private physician who consults a colleague about a case and indicates that "his" student found a certain physical finding will have a devoted student forever—as will the teacher who mentions to his office nurse the generally good work that a resident is doing, or the teacher who mentions to a patient, with the student present, what a pleasure it is to have such a good student in the office. This is not actual positive feedback nor does it give blanket approval to all the learner's actions but it does build a reservoir of goodwill upon which to draw in the future if the teacher needs to give unpleasant but important negative feedback.

Love notes. These are private demonstrations of the same general support and goodwill described above. The attending physician assigned to an inpatient team, the faculty team leader of an ambulatory care team, and student/resident advisors can provide encouragement and support by sending learners briefly written but generally positive comments. Jotting a friendly note on a reprint that might be of interest to a resident or passing along positive comments heard second-hand are good rapport builders.

6. Surface Paraphrasing and Exploration

Surface paraphrasing and exploration are the transition from attentive silence to cooperative negotiation. The teacher using these skills wants more information from the student but wants him to delve deeper himself, without the teacher taking a major negotiating position or requesting in-depth discussions. When a student stumbles to a halt in the middle of presenting a patient with respiratory distress of unknown cause, the teacher might say, "You seem unclear whether to pursue cardiac or pulmonary causes for this problem." When a student on a psychiatric rotation presents a somatizing patient whose symptoms seem to jump from one organ system to another, the teacher can clarify the situation by asking, "It seems that the patient is unclear why he really came here today?" Of course, the student is even less clear why the patient came, but reflecting on the patient's confusion is a supportive way of suggesting the student's own uncertainty. Other helpful questions are derived from patient-interviewing training: "So you think that you need to admit this patient now?" "You seem to be focusing a lot on this patient's headache?" "Tell me again about the indications for surgery in ulcer patients." Exploratory questions can sometimes be asked tentatively so that the learner can pass over them quickly if he wishes. At other times the "digging" is more serious, which leads the teacher into more active skills described in the next section. In either case, paraphrasing and exploration help gather additional facts, help to look at more sides of a situation, or emphasize the areas of importance and interest to both teacher and learner.

Cooperative Negotiation

Negotiation between teacher and learner suggests the coming together of equals—an adult-adult relationship in which the teacher and learner each have needs and expectations that are worthy and require negotiation if discrepant. As previously noted, this notion of equals is not always appreciated in medical education settings, where the marked differences between teacher and learner in knowledge and experience often resembles those of a parent-child relationship. However, depth of knowledge and experience is only one of the "issues" brought to the "negotiating table." The other areas requiring negotiation are needs, expectations, and roles (Pratt & Magill 1983).

Learner needs usually include the desire to learn, to be proficient, to be successful, and to please the teacher. Teacher needs include the desire to be helpful, to demonstrate competence, to influence the learner's behavior, and to assure the competence of the learner. These sets of needs are equally worthy and deserve similar consideration in any negotiations between equals. Expectations are equally worthy in both parties: The teacher expects that the learner will work hard, be well-meaning, and be considerate of the teacher's needs; the learner expects that the learning will be valuable, the teacher will be considerate, and the learning climate reasonable and constructive. The roles brought to the negotiation by teacher and learner are most discrepant and likely to lead to conflict. Teachers can play one or more of several roles (Mann et al. 1970; see chapter 3) including that of expert, socializing agent, facilitator, ego ideal, and person. Note that only one of these roles is that of expert, which, by virtue of greater experience and knowledge, puts the teacher in a far superior position to that of the learner. The learner can also play one of several roles, including that of compliant student, the anxious-dependent student and the sniper (see chapter 3). Pratt and Magill (1983) describe three different sorts of roles: the dependent, competitive, or participant students. The latter two are those in which the student acts most nearly equal to the teacher, but even dependent roles have to be negotiated from a position of equality. The senior resident who still approaches the attending, even as graduation approaches, wanting to "dump" a hard patient problem on the teacher should not be offered the role of dependency, with the teacher as expert, regardless of the learner's expectations.

The following behaviors and skills will help the teacher approach the learner on a more nearly equal basis.

7. Self-Disclosure

One of the easiest techniques with which to effectively deal with learners as equals is for the teacher to disclose personal information: feelings, professional attitudes, past experiences (either personal or professional), "war stories," and mistakes. Some teachers are not comfortable doing this and perhaps never will. Many teachers have a considerable fear of revealing anything personal to learners, particularly inadequacies in professional competence, because of the notion that teachers must appear all knowing and infallible. Physician readers will recognize this attitude as one that prevailed in physician-patient relationships in the past—a paternalistic omnipotent concept of the God-like physician caring for the passive-dependent patient. This notion has undergone remarkable transformation recently (Katz 1985), and this same new physician self-concept applies in the situation of the physician as teacher. The paradox of the teacher-learner relationship is that learners view teachers as more experienced when they reveal errors, more knowledgeable when they admit deficiencies, more powerful when they reveal weaknesses, and more influential when they say "I don't know." Of course, as is true for too much of anything, an excess of professional humility can also be a problem. On the whole, however, most physician teachers would benefit from humbly revealing their humanity to their learners, especially since learners have known all along that teachers are people too. Here are four examples:

1. When a case discussion on teaching rounds ends with a difficult question whose answer will not immediately affect the treatment that the team will be providing the patient the attending can say, "I don't know the best answer for that, but I'll look it up and bring some ideas to rounds tomorrow." Assigning the investigation to a student or resident is even more effective.

2. When a student is asked a question by an ambulatory patient that the student cannot answer and the attending is also unable to answer, the physician teacher can tell the student, "I don't know," in front of the patient; the teacher can also provide a plan for finding out the answer to the patient's question. This is not only good self-disclosure but rescues the student from the patient's potential feelings of dissatisfaction with the student's care.

3. A resident's feelings of frustration and dejection with a case that has had a bad outcome are most effectively handled by the attending physician revealing similar feelings and describing similar cases with bad outcomes. Seeing an experienced physician share memories of adversity, yet demonstrating that his career and successes obviously continued, is a powerful educational experience for learners. Similar sharing of situations causing anxiety (e.g., first time running a "code", first testimony in a courtroom), sadness (e.g., making a diagnosis of cancer in a child, telling a young wife that her husband has died of a myocardial infarction), or elation (e.g., delivering one's first baby, receiving a present or note of thanks from a patient) are equally effective.

4. Simply repeating a learner's expressed feelings in an empathic way is a form of self-disclosure since the teacher suggests that he may have felt or thought similarly: "You seem to be feeling pretty badly that Mrs. Smith died?" "Are you worried about whether the child with croup will make it through the night without mist treatment?" "I hear from the chief resident that you're having quite a time deciding between private practice and an HMO job next year."

8. Active Listening

The last example above is a blend between self-disclosure and active listening, since the teacher is asking questions that are designed to expand upon a simple statement made by the learner. The term *active listening* suggests that an opposite, *passive listening,* may also exist. This is true, and has been described previously as *open-ended encouragement* and *surface paraphrasing.* These last two teacher behaviors are gentle probings that reflect back to what the learner has just said or done. Active listening, on the other hand, is a more active probing whose purpose is clarification, expansion, justification, and correlation. The teacher uses something the learner has just said or done (usually said) as a starting point and with mild questioning attempts to expand the learner's thinking:

1. (Use in a lecture setting.) "Are you asking whether visual changes are a part of digitalis toxicity?"
2. "Tell me more about the heart murmur you just mentioned."
3. "You mentioned before that the patient had no previous breathing problems. How does that relate to the aminophylline you just said he is taking?"
4. "Tell me again about the neurologic spell you said she had?"
5. "I still don't understand exactly why she came to the ER today?"

9. Intense Paraphrasing

On the active-passive spectrum of behavior, intense paraphrasing is the next most active behavior after active listening and is much more forceful than surface paraphrasing. Intense paraphrasing suggests that the intent is more aggressive or assertive, that the purpose is more defined, and that the desired response or information is more specific. The teacher is more focused and is obviously probing deeper. This behavior is not as intense or probing as the more confrontational techniques described in the next section, but the teacher is far more assertive than in previous, more passive, situations. Here are four examples, from both classroom and clinical teaching:

1. "You mentioned before that the patient's chief complaint is pain in the flank and costovertebral angle, but now you're going into detail about the patient's cardiac risk factors. Could you clarify that discrepancy for us?"

2. "In a previous session you made a joke about alcoholics, and now you seem to be saying that we should discontinue further treatment for the patient in this case discussion. Could you elaborate on why you think that?"

3. "Tell us more about the indications for surgery in ulcer disease, especially the issue of intractable pain you mentioned just briefly."

4. "You started to tell us the factors that are associated with child abuse. Please continue on, focusing on parental behavior at the time of the child's delivery."

10. Open-Ended Questioning

Open-end questioning may seem a less confrontational or assertive technique than intense paraphrasing, but actually is more stimulating. The reader will notice that the examples given in the sections on surface paraphrasing, active listening, and intense paraphrasing were fairly direct and focused questions. The teacher was asking questions about specific subjects that were usually raised by the student or resident. The questions were asked in a way that directed the learner's thinking quite specifically. The teacher had a specific agenda, both for the subject of the question and for the direction that he wished the learner to take. These closed questions serve specific and valuable purposes, but they do not open the learner's thinking as much as open-ended questions. When using open-ended questions, the teacher usually wishes to expand the learner's thinking rather than narrow it to one or a few choices or ideas.

Open-ended questioning has several valuable educational purposes, whereas closed questioning is only used to ascertain whether the learner knows a particular answer or fact. The technique of questioning has, among others, the following uses (Schwenk & Whitman 1984):

1. To stimulate learning and thinking;
2. To assist the learner in organizing and clarifying concepts;
3. To correct misunderstandings or faulty reasoning (right answer but wrong reason);
4. To assist in showing special or obscure relationships;
5. To strengthen the learner's ability to synthesize and analyze;
6. To correct attitudes or behavior.

Types of questions that promote this type of critical thinking are those that are open ended and divergent. Students should be asked to clarify, support, defend, justify, correlate, critique, evaluate, analyze, interpret, and predict. They should not be asked to regurgitate facts or answers with one or a few words. During medical case presentations, for example (see chapter 7), the following are examples of questions that can be used to stimulate problem solving and critical thinking:

1. "At this point in the presentation, what hypotheses do you have in mind?"
2. "Why did you just ask _____ ?"
3. "Based on the historical information presented, what physical examination findings will be particularly important to note?"
4. "What is your evaluation of the previous medical care received by this patient?"
5. "If [*physical examination finding*] were present [*absent*] instead of absent [*present*], how would it change your differential diagnosis?"
6. "What further laboratory data might clarify the differential diagnosis?"
7. "If [*laboratory test*] were positive [*negative*] instead of negative [*positive*], how would it change your differential diagnosis?"
8. "What would you do if [*laboratory test*] were unavailable?"
9. "What are the most likely diagnoses?"
10. "What pieces of information tend to support your best hypothesis?"
11. "What pieces of information tend to detract from your best hypothesis?"
12. "Critique the treatment plan proposed by [*another student or resident*]."
13. "Do you think this patient should be [*have been*] admitted to the hospital? Why or why not?"

Similar questions can be asked in other settings, such as lectures when rhetorical questions are asked, and in group discussions when this style of questioning is the norm:

1. "If I were to ask you to analyze this set of arterial blood gases shown on the slide, what would you say about the arterial-alveolar gradient?"

2. "Here is a set of abnormal serum electrolytes. What would you do about them?"
3. "Compare these two slides of normal and cirrhotic liver parenchyma."

11. Giving Positive and Negative Feedback

Although the term *feedback* was first used by rocket engineers in the 1940s (Whitman 1985), "feedback" now is used in the context of human performance. Feedback is the process of giving learners information about current performance so that they may improve it in the future. Giving feedback is the most assertive thing a physician-teacher can do short of moving into a more confrontational mode of interacting with learners (as described in the next section). Feedback can be either positive or negative. Positive feedback is given to reinforce good behavior, and negative feedback to change bad behavior. It is therefore easy to confuse positive feedback with compliments and negative feedback with criticism. Generally, neither of these associations is pertinent to the use of feedback by physician-teachers. Compliments are aimed at making the "receiver" feel better, and criticisms are aimed at making the "giver" feel better—neither is designed to help improve performance. The feedback that teachers should use in medical education is information, judgments, or observations that help the student or resident make improvements.

Many guidelines for giving feedback have been suggested for medical educators (e.g., Berquist & Phillips 1975; Ende 1983). Three characteristics of feedback are common to the two sets of guidelines just cited. First, feedback should be *descriptive* rather than *evaluative*. For example, during an observed physical examination, a medical student has difficulty using the ophthalmoscope. An evaluative statement by the teacher would be, "You're really clumsy." A better form of feedback would be a descriptive statement, such as, "The patient appeared anxious when you were having trouble using the ophthalmoscope." Descriptive feedback is more helpful because it provides an unambiguous and relatively unarguable point from which to start suggesting ways for improvement.

Second, feedback should be as specific as possible. For example, a resident hears a benign systolic ejection murmur in a woman whose father has died of a myocardial infarction. The resident carefully explains the significant differences between the two conditions, and the teacher wishes to comment positively on this behavior. A general statement such as, "I've noticed that you are very sensitive to patient concerns," is a nice compliment but does little to reinforce the resident's specific behavior that was so reassuring to the patient. A more helpful and specific statement would be, "I noticed that, when you explained the difference between the patient's benign heart murmur and her father's atherosclerotic heart disease, you seemed to relieve an unspoken concern of hers."

Third, feedback should be "well timed," meaning that it should be delivered as soon after the event or behavior as is reasonable and practical. In fast-paced clinical settings, feedback more than a few days old is "old news" and has far less impact on future performance than if delivered immediately. Physician teachers are familiar with the typical evaluation of medical students, which students see months after a course or rotation, when students or residents not only cannot adjust their behavior in response to the feedback but cannot even remember their previous performance. However, there may be times when feedback immediately after the event is neither possible nor desirable. If either party does not have time, feedback that is rushed or forced may not be effective. Also, if either the teacher or learner is very upset after some poor performance or adverse outcome, which is often the case when negative feedback is warranted, then the ability to either give or receive feedback effectively is impaired. If the feedback is negative or personal issues are discussed, it may be better to give it in a private and comfortable setting, which may be a scarce commodity in most clinical teaching settings or in large, impersonal medical student lectures. If feedback is worth giving, it should be done well, unless the only purpose for doing so is to make the "giver" feel better, in which case it is merely criticism.

When giving negative feedback that is of particularly critical or sensitive, some teachers think it is better to give some positive feedback first, then to follow the negative feedback with some more positive comments. "Tell 'em what was good, tell 'em what was not good, and tell 'em again what was good." This approach fails when "what was good" was also trivial and not relevant to the learner's overall performance. For example, if a student doing a preceptorship in a private practice has been rude to the office staff, this approach would trivialize the important negative feedback: "John, I would like to talk with you about your first few days here in my office. First of all, I would like you to know how much I appreciate your clean-cut, well-groomed appearance. However, an area of your performance that disturbs me is the way you chastised and insulted my head office nurse. However, I like your neat handwriting in the charts."

The problem with beginning with positive feedback when the intent is to give negative feedback is that usually the learner can detect a ring of insincerity. The lack of authenticity often is apparent and can actually make giving and receiving negative feedback more stressful than usual. When the good parts, the "bread" of the good-bad-good "sandwich," are trivial, it becomes a bologna sandwich.

A solution for this dilemma is to develop a reservoir of goodwill as soon as possible in a relationship with a learner, so that negative feedback can be given in a pure form, yet with a cushion of good past experiences to soften the blow. This is the approach suggested by Blanchard and Johnson's (1982) *The One-Minute Manager*. Giving someone positive feedback as soon as it is truly deserved creates a history that allows the learner to receive negative feedback constructively, without having it sandwiched between contrived positive statements.

The straightforward approach, without a reservoir of goodwill, can sometimes generate defensiveness and hostility. Occasionally, physician teachers will have a learner who becomes defensive even when all the guidelines are followed, probably because of bad past experiences that have nothing to do with that particular teacher. In this situation, the teacher might give feedback regarding that person's ability to accept negative feedback: "I noticed that when I tried to give you some feedback regarding your workup of that patient, you seemed to become hostile. I felt that you were putting your energy into defending your actions, instead of trying to make use of what I was telling you. I tried to be descriptive and specific, so that what I had to say about your workup would be helpful. I'm concerned, because I feel as if I have given you positive feedback when deserved, but that you don't seem able to use negative feedback. How do you see this situation?"

Asking the learner for his opinion about his performance is almost always a helpful technique, and the educational research suggests that self-evaluation is probably the most powerful type of evaluation possible. This approach insures that the teacher has a more complete view of the situation and might obviate the need to give painful negative feedback that the learner already understands. In this case, the discussion can then focus on how the learner can make use of the knowledge of his performance he already has.

Another reason for soliciting learner information and understanding "where the learner is at" is that often students may be wrong for the right reasons, or right for the wrong reasons. Physician teachers giving feedback, whether positive or negative, without accurate information or background run several risks: They may be rewarding a superficially correct answer that the learner does not fundamentally understand, the teacher may be met with defensiveness, the teacher may lose the effectiveness of the feedback by confusion and debate over "the facts of the case," or the teacher may have difficulty in ever effectively giving feedback to that learner again because of lost credibility. As a humorous example, Klass (1985) relates the story of the attending physician who presented to his ward team the case of a patient admitted through the emergency room with severe low back pain. The case was very complex and confusing, but after its presentation, the attending asked his students for their diagnoses, assuming they would be quite wrong. One student, without hesitation, suggested a leaking or ruptured aortic aneurysm. The attending was astounded—that was the correct diagnosis! The attending then asked for a further clarification of the student's thinking that led to that diagnosis. The student replied, "So what else causes lower back pain?"

More seriously, physician faculty are often asked to intercede with students or residents whose behavior or performance is considered deficient by faculty or other residents. This deficient performance may take the form of mistakes in writing orders, poor patient follow-up or patient relationships, irresponsible behavior on other services, poor interprofessional relationships, or other unprofessional behavior that the physician-teacher has not witnessed directly. In these situations, an understanding of the learner's perceptions is critical so that a balanced judgment and assessment can be made. The "two sides to every story" cliche is never more true than here. An understanding of both sides is necessary for a successful confrontation.

Persuasive Confrontation

The third, and final, set of interaction skills concerns the most assertive posture that the teacher can adopt—persuasive confrontation. This set of skills parallels the role of the physician who takes control of a patient interview or patient relationship and who is active in controlling the pace of the interaction and its outcome. For the physician teacher, this means adopting what was previously considered the *only* role of a medical teacher, that of expert. As has been shown, there are many other possible roles, but with the skills that follow, the teacher is clearly superior in knowledge and experience and is transmitting this to the learner. For example, in a study of family practice residents in Ohio (Wolverton & Bosworth 1985), at least 6 of 38 moderately to extremely helpful teaching behaviors that were studied required an assertive teacher role:

1. Defines realistic learning objectives;
2. Directs residents to useful references in the literature;
3. Identifies resident's strengths/weaknesses objectively;
4. Presents teaching points in a well-organized manner;
5. Logically explains basis for actions/decisions;
6. Corrects mistakes without belittling.

Interestingly, the last behavior was rated by the residents as most helpful of the entire group of 38 behaviors. The types of behaviors included in this section on persuasive confrontation include summarizing, interpreting, information giving, prescribing, critiquing, correcting, closed questioning, persuading, and challenging and confronting.

12. Summarizing and Interpreting

Summarizing and interpreting are the least confrontational of this last set of behaviors. For learners, they are the most benign way for the teacher to take charge of the interaction. The teacher has control of the subject being discussed and can add appropriate emphasis, clarity, or emotional punctuation. A standard lecture is actually a summary and interpretation of a body of knowledge. A summary at the end of a small group discussion, such as a journal club or weekly student topic conference, is an extremely effective way of closing a stimulating discussion. Similarly, a highly participative hallway discussion of a case may raise several issues, such as alternative diagnoses or possible treatment approaches. A concluding summary by the attending clarifies those findings, diagnoses, or treatments most worthy of confirmation or consideration and clarifies what will happen next, or who is to do what next:

1. "What I have heard so far is that irritable bowel syndrome, peptic ulcer disease, and cholecystitis are all possible diagnoses. I feel most strongly that this is cholecystitis, and that we should do an ultrasound of the gallbladder next."

2. "In summary, I have presented several treatment approaches for migraine headaches. You have asked a number of questions about biofeedback approaches, which I think is an important topic, and we will talk about that next time."

3. "What you're telling me is that this patient is not as sick as his private doctor thought, and the patient doesn't need to be in the hospital. I tend to agree with that, although you mentioned this questionable history of weight loss over the past three months that requires clarification."

4. "What I'm hearing is a story of a patient with longstanding chronic obstructive lung disease who probably needs to be on home oxygen for comfort reasons, even though the arterial blood gases that you presented are somewhat borderline."

13. Information Giving and Prescribing

These behaviors are exactly parallel to those used with a patient. Physicians prescribe for patients, both with medications and with advice. They also are constantly giving information, about preventing disease or about the features and consequences of disease already present. Physicians are powerful patient educators, and that power extends to giving information and prescribing to learners. In fact, the same characteristics of effective patient education apply to giving information to learners (Dodge 1983; Ley et al. 1976):

Limit the amount of information given. Contrary to popular opinion in medical education, more is rarely better. As described in more detail in chapter 5 (Lectures), the most effective method of transmitting information is to give a moderate amount, neither too little nor too much (e.g., about 8–10 important facts in a 1-hour lecture). Too many facts become obscured such that fewer are retained, while too few give the learner too little to work with. In an interesting parallel between patient care and teaching, research by Ley and Spellman (1965) showed that eight or more facts given to a patient are likely to overload the patient, such that at least four facts will be forgotten.

Give the most important facts first. Teachers who begin with obscure and tangential facts may never have the opportunity to move to the critical and fundamental information. Labeling the most important facts as such is also helpful. Some teachers still consider hiding the important facts (e.g., those to be asked in test questions) as a valid teaching technique, as if a high level of information retention by the student were somehow a bad outcome—an attitude we hope will rapidly go the way of inkwells and hickory switches.

Stress the importance of the instructions or information to the learner's needs. If the teacher cannot clarify the importance of the material, why should the learner listen?

Avoid jargon. This is an equal problem for patients and medical students, and students may feel even more inhibited about asking for clarification than patients. Students may understand actual terms, but may be very confused about underlying concepts and principles. When the teacher is in a "telling mode," rather than in a listening or questioning stance, the burden is on the teacher to somehow check the learner's understanding, either at that time or at a defined later time.

Relate information clearly to the problem at hand. There may be appropriate times for giving background information, whose use is not immediately apparent, but the burden is on the teacher to demonstrate the value of doing so. Students, and, even more so, residents, are very task oriented and are anxious to learn information that will help solve an immediate problem. Whether this attitude is right or wrong, the teacher must relate each fact to the problem or patient of concern and must make the relevance clear.

Use repetition for emphasis. The teacher repeating information, directives, or assignments reinforces the material's importance and allows the learner to check his understanding. Having the learner repeat the information is even more effective. Simply asking patients to repeat the physician's instructions increased the patients' recall of the information by 20% in one study (Bertakis 1977). The effect on learners should be at least as great.

Make instructions specific, behavioral, and measurable. This suggestion refers to directions given by the physician teacher to a learner to carry out a certain assignment. The learner must go away from that interaction knowing not only what the outcome of his activity should be (e.g., "We need to get the stool tested for occult blood.") but how the goal is to be accomplished (e.g., "Do a rectal exam right now and test the specimen yourself."). Otherwise, the learner may devise other, less acceptable methods (e.g., "I wrote an order for a stool gauaic test. We should receive the results in about 3 days.").

Present alternately acceptable treatments or procedures. Just as patients do well when given some choices in their instructions, learners benefit when they must choose between equally acceptable approaches to a patient or problem. The increased feelings of control and involvement markedly increase learning (Rogers 1951).

In summary, the traditional role of the teacher is telling learners how to think and what to do. As described earlier in this chapter, there are actually many other ways for teachers to teach besides "instructing," but when telling, giving information, and prescribing are useful, the eight steps just described help make that active role more effective. Here are four examples of giving information or prescribing:

1. "We've heard several possible diagnostic approaches. Here are the three most important things I want you to do first. Then we'll see which approach seems to be headed in the right direction."

2. "The lecture today is on the interpretation of arterial blood gases. This information is critical to your ability to care for the patients you'll see on your upcoming pulmonary medicine rotation." Early in the lecture: "Here are the six points we'll cover today . . . ."

Later in the lecture: "The fifth important point is . . . ." Towards the end of the lecture: "Here are the six steps we covered today in how to interpret arterial blood gases." This is an example of the old educational aphorism, "Tell 'em what you're going to tell 'em, tell 'em, then tell 'em what you told 'em."

3. "This is a handout on the interpretation of maternal alpha-fetoprotein assays. Does everyone understand what this test is and the diseases in which it is used?"

4. "I think it would be equally acceptable to do either an upper GI series or gastroscopy. Which do you want to do?"

14. Critiquing, Correcting, and Closed Questioning

These behaviors are just short of being the most assertive way a teacher can behave toward a student. Critiquing and correcting are in a sense giving feedback, but more for the purpose of evaluation than for helping the learner improve. In the evaluation model used by Scriven (1967), the giving of feedback is a type of *formative evaluation* used for the purpose of improving future performance, while critiquing and correcting the learner and asking closed questions to elicit short answers is a type of *summative evaluation* that is primarily a judgment of competence.

Closed questions are those that can be briefly answered with a "yes," "no," or a short phrase. The information obtained is very focused, and these questions are convergent, meaning that they narrow the range of information under discussion, rather than expanding the discussion by being divergent. As in the use of closed questions with patients, the information obtained is very specific, therefore the question has to be quite precise, asking just what the teacher wants to know. This is similarly true with critiquing and correcting a student, in which the teacher has to be very accurate and specific in the comments so as to pinpoint areas of deficiency without being personally demeaning or extending the criticism to behaviors or knowledge that are actually correct. Leading questions are at the least unhelpful and at the most counterproductive, since the learner feels exploited or manipulated and the information elicited is likely to be contaminated by the teacher's biases. Here are four examples of how learners may be critiqued, corrected, or questioned in a closed and direct fashion:

1. "I understand why you think this abnormality on the chest x-ray represents a pneumonia, but you are wrong. Here's why."
2. "Tell me what you think we should do about this low serum potassium level?"
3. "I observed you talking to that patient's daughter, and you were quite abrupt and rude. That behavior is unacceptable."
4. "You described minimal pharyngeal erythema and no tonsillar erythema or pus for this patient with a sore throat. Why did you prescribe antibiotics?"

15. Persuasion, Challenge, and Confrontation

The most assertive teacher behavior is to confront a learner about previously held attitudes or knowledge and persuade him to change them in some way. This is the most difficult but perhaps the ultimate objective for any teacher-learner interaction. Confrontation is useful in patients who are unmotivated to change a behavior, whose compliance is poor, or who have personality disorders or substance abuse problems that prevent an effective physician-patient relationship or who are particularly reserved or repressed in their communications. Some of these conditions apply in teaching situations where learners are particularly intransigent in learning new knowledge, attitudes, or skills; seem resistant or unmotivated; or have ineffective learning habits. Hopefully, these will be infrequent situations, but command of these skills is still essential for a master physician teacher.

Effective confrontation is based on the use of "I" messages, meaning that the teacher bases the confrontation on his personal feelings or beliefs and how the learner is affecting those feelings or beliefs. Effective "I" messages have the following characteristics:

1. They do not reduce, but rather preserve, the learner's self-esteem.
2. They state the teacher's feelings clearly and congruently, however strong they may be, in a way that the teacher truly feels.
3. They leave the possible solutions to the learner, so as to preserve student autonomy.
4. They lead to a logical conclusion, rather than appearing as isolated accusations out of context.
5. They often require active work by the teacher to deal with the learner's emotional reaction.

The teacher can phrase the message to include three elements: a description of the specific offending behavior or attitude that is not blameful; a statement of how that behavior is a problem, incorrect, or otherwise unacceptable to the teacher; and a description of why it is unacceptable. Here are some examples:

1. "You have asked that same question for the last three lectures. When you do that, I feel very upset, because I think my lecture must be unhelpful. Is that true?"

2. "When you are rude to the office nurse, I get worried because if you do that in your future practice, you may have significant office staff problems. I also get angry because it causes our office staff here to become dissatisfied, which may affect the quality of our patient care."

3. "When you continue to dress and care for yourself in such an unprofessional manner, I get angry because it reflects badly on the entire training program."

4. "When you tell me you're going to pull the patient's Foley catheter, and then don't do it, I feel upset that you may be disagreeing with the plan, but aren't telling me."

5. "We agreed that you would prepare this report by today. Now that I see it's not done, I feel angry, because the extra time I have put into working with you seems to have been wasted."

Summary

This chapter described 15 behaviors or teaching skills that form a rich repertoire for the physician teacher. Literally everything that a teacher does is on or derived in some way from this list. Both classroom and clinical teaching draw on this set of behaviors. The list is a continuum that spans the most passive to the most assertive ways in which a teacher can behave with a learner. The 15 types of behavior are derived directly from related behaviors that a physician might use with a patient. The physician teacher is already experienced with these corresponding patient interviewing behaviors and should find their translation to teaching relatively easy. Methods of directly applying these behaviors to all types of teaching are described in part II.

The Five Teaching Responsibilities of the Physician

Part Two presents specific and practical guidelines to help faculty members become good teachers in didactic and clinical settings. Each chapter addresses a particular setting with a brief introduction followed by a discussion of objectives, techniques, and tips. The authors' aim is to direct the attention of physician readers to the application of the communication skills described in Part One.

CHAPTER 5

Lectures

A medical school professor is lecturing to a virtually empty classroom and a
spinning tape recorder. As the talk ends, one of the few students present
retrieves the recorder and prepares to transcribe the lecture and to distribute
copies to classmates who stayed away (Altman 1982).

According to Dr. Lawrence K. Altman, the medical editor for *The
New York Times*, the above story is not apocryphal. In his visits to
several medical schools, students told him it occurs because they
believe they are studying more efficiently by cutting boring lectures
and using that time to read textbooks and transcripts of lectures. The
same story was repeated by Dr. Ludwig Eichna, who returned to
medical school as a student after retiring from the chairmanship of
the Department of Medicine at the State University of New York,
Downstate Medical Center. After completing all four years of medical
school, Eichna (1980, p. 729) decried the emphasis on the accumulation of facts:

> Ingrained by previous schooling with the habit of getting the
> facts to pass the examinations, students stay away from
> thinking activities. Instead lecturers find a student's tape re-
> corder in the front row. The "student syndicate" has the
> lectures transcribed, typed, and sold to students, who stay

home to study the transcripts, for the examinations are based on lecture facts.

The problem with medical school lectures was highlighted further by Dr. David E. Rogers (1982, p. 11), President of The Robert Wood Johnson Foundation, who was told by medical students that they felt they were being "lectured to death". In addition to the personal criticism leveled at medical lectures by these physician educators, a more official censure appeared in the recently publicized report on the General Professional Education of the Physician [(GPEP) Association of American Medical Colleges 1984]. According to the GPEP report, although lecturing is the predominant method of instruction in medical schools, there is abundant evidence that its educational yield is generally low.

According to the editors of *Change Magazine* (1978), the lecture is the major medium of instruction in higher education and the most abused; apparently this is true in medical education as well. However, although lectures are in disrepute, we believe that they can be quite effective when used properly and for the appropriate objectives.

Objectives

There are two proper uses of the lecture: To present information that does not appear in print, or that appears in print but has been synthesized from many sources. Information that does not appear in print includes unpublished research findings; however, probably the most important medical information of that kind is a physician's own clinical experience. The use of unpublished findings and personal experiences makes students and residents aware of a medical educator as both a teacher and a physician; therefore we encourage this role modeling as much as possible.

With regard to the second use of lectures, providing a synthesis of information that appears in print is a valuable use of medical teachers. Of course, if learners did the synthesis themselves, they probably would learn more than from a lecture. Realistically, residents and, especially, medical students, may lack the time or ability to synthesize the material. In this case, we support using a lecture to synthesize printed material for them.

If information presented in a lecture can be read in a book, we question whether this is a proper use of the lecture. Would not students be better off reading the material on their own and at their own pace? We think so, especially in the light of the principles of adult learning discussed in earlier chapters. Perhaps the reader now is wondering, "If it is better to let adults read on their own, then perhaps the student transcription services described by Altman (1982) and Eichna (1980) should be encouraged. In fact, should medical teachers write out their lectures and not lecture at all?" That was precisely the recommendation made in B. F. Skinner's utopian novel, *Walden Two* (1948), where lecturing to students was characterized as "platform chicanery." Why not hand out printed lectures to students as suggested by Skinner?

The reason this is not a good idea lies in the fact that, in addition to conveying information, a lecture can present information with an emotional impact. According to Foley and Smilansky (1980, p. 5) summaries of research on teaching consistently cite the importance of warmth and enthusiasm. They conclude that "these traits are as important in the lecture as in teaching situations that involve more direct interaction with the students."

Thus, the lecture provides medical teachers with opportunities to convey their personal interest in the subject. One creative teacher emphasized the need to provide the "inner relevance" of a subject (Kestin 1970), and another spoke of instruction as a two-part process, "presenting information while at the same time indicating its worth" (Ericksen 1980, p. 5). Emotional impact is what makes a lecture different, and better, than a transcript; the teacher's enthusiasm makes students feel that the subject is valuable and worth knowing. According to the jargon of instructional technology, this is an example of an *affective* objective. Affective objectives seek to influence the learner's feelings, values, or attitudes. So, "this subject is worth knowing" is an example of an affective objective, which we think is an appropriate generic objective for every medical lecture.

What about other affective objectives? Is it appropriate to use a lecture to try to change more specific feelings, values, or attitudes? In general, we think not. When there is a specific affective objective, such as "chronic pain should not be confused with symptom faking and malingering," we recommend the group discussion method, which will be addressed in the next chapter.

The problem with trying to achieve specific affective objectives in a lecture is that it can sound like a sermon. For the most part, the appropriate objectives for a lecture are *cognitive*. In other words, there is information not known by learners at the start of a lecture that they will know at the end. According to Bloom et al. (1956), there are six levels of cognitive objectives:

1. Knowledge;
2. Comprehension;
3. Application;
4. Analysis;
5. Synthesis;
6. Evaluation.

At the lowest level, there are knowledge objectives, which require remembering new facts. At one level higher, there are comprehension objectives, which require understanding what the facts mean. Knowledge and comprehension objectives can be achieved in a lecture, i.e., learners leave the lecture knowing and understanding things they did not know and understand before the lecture. As is true of all instructional objectives, knowledge and comprehension are measured in terms of learner outcomes. Earlier, we cited as an example of a specific affective objective, "chronic pain should not be confused with symptom faking and malingering." This is not a realistic objective for a lecture, i.e., a teacher will not change many views with a lecture. However, in a lecture on chronic pain, there are some realistic knowledge and comprehension objectives, e.g., as a result of the lecture, students will be able to compare and contrast radiating versus referred pain.

The third level of cognitive objectives concerns *application, i.e.,* using information in new ways. For example, in the lecture on chronic pain, after presenting information on "mislocations of pain," the teacher could ask students in class to use the information in the following situation:

> As a result of a truck accident, a man has chronic, deep pain in the upper margin of the scapula and numbness along the ulnar side of the forearm and hand. When a local anesthetic was injected in the area of deep pain, normal pain sensation returned to the forearm and hand. How can this be explained?

While all lectures should aim at achieving knowledge and comprehension objectives, aiming at application objectives is optional. If application is the aim of a lecture, the teacher should provide an opportunity for the students to actually use the information. For some lectures, achievement of application objectives may not be possible or desirable, depending upon the level of the learners. What about the three successively higher levels of objectives: analysis (breaking a subject down into its parts), synthesis (putting the parts together in a new way), and evaluation (making judgments about the subject)? Realistically, these objectives cannot be achieved in a lecture. At best, a teacher can *model* those higher level cognitive objectives, but learners have to be more actively involved than is possible in a lecture. These higher-level objectives will be addressed in the next chapter on group discussion.

Thus far, we have discussed affective and cognitive objectives. The third domain, *psychomotor* or *skill* objectives, cannot be achieved in a lecture. Psychomotor or skill objectives are more appropriate in the "application" environment of clinical teaching, i.e., preceptorships and tutorials. Occasionally, a lecture orientation to a new skill, e.g., how to interview a patient, is helpful. However, student frustration and boredom will soon appear if an instructor attempts to actually teach a skill in a lecture format. We are reminded of the teacher who began a lecture about reading:

> Children, today I am going to teach you *all* about reading. Listen carefully, because I have some important things to tell you about reading. Ronald, close that book! How are you ever going to learn to read if you keep looking at books!

Techniques

Teachers may know the proper use of lecturing and what objectives are appropriate and realistic, but not *how* to lecture. The key to making an effective lecture presentation lies in the use of teaching techniques that attract and maintain attention.

Attracting attention is important because learners walk into a classroom with many different concerns and priorities, some of which have nothing to do with the subject of the lecture. The reason why a lecturer wants to attract attention is to focus the minds of the learners on the subject to be presented. One technique to attract attention is to tell a relevant anecdote. David R. Mouw (1980), who taught physiology at the University of Michigan Medical School, has described an anecdote he used to get across the principle that urine is essentially composed, not of waste products, but rather of water and salt, which are present in the body in excess. The anecdote he told was of his honeymoon, when he and his wife took a canoe trip in a wilderness area of Michigan's Upper Peninsula. Due to the hordes of mosquitos, they did not want to leave their tent at night once they got into it. They wanted to empty their bladders, but the only available container was their coffee pot. Knowing there was nothing harmful in urine, except maybe a few bacteria from the urethral orifice that would be easily killed by boiling, they used their coffee pot to empty their bladders at night and to brew coffee in the morning.

In order to decide when to use an anecdote, Mouw has established five criteria, which we recommend to all lecturers:

1. The anecdote must illustrate a principle he is trying to teach.
2. Listening to it must be enjoyable.
3. The anecdote should be personal, telling the students something about the teacher as a person.
4. Students should be able to relate to the situation described.
5. It is nice if the anecdote is funny, but that is not essential.

A second technique to attract attention is to pose a dilemma or raise an issue which the lecture will later address. For example, to attract attention at the start of the chronic pain lecture, the teacher might tell the "pain game" (Posner 1984, p. 60):

> Patient: "I hurt. Please fix me (but you cannot)."
> Doctor: "I will fix you."

> After multiple diagnostic procedures, which often do not elicit the exact etiology of the patient's pain and may involve several referrals to consultants, the patient may still have pain. The pain transaction is then completed when the patient returns to the physician and the following exchange occurs:

> Patient (with righteous indignation): "Another incompetent quack."
> Doctor (defensively): "Another crock."

Other techniques to attract attention include surveying the audience (e.g., "How many of you have chronic pain?"), asking a rhetorical question, and reading a controversial quotation. The major principle is that a teacher wants to focus learners on the subject, get them thinking, and begin the process of mental engagement. Using techniques to attract attention provides teachers with many opportunities to be creative.

Creativity also is needed to maintain attention. Because of the passive role of learners in a lecture, their attention span is relatively short. The loss of attention in 15–20 minutes was noted in the research on college teaching reviewed by Davis and Alexander (1977) and in a study of medical students by Stuart and Rutherford (1978). Thus, we recommend that teachers use a technique to help maintain attention at the 15–20 minute mark of their lectures. The use of such a technique may use 5–10 minutes of a lecture and should be considered a worthwhile investment of time. As stated by McKeachie (1965, p. 22), "One of the problems of the lecturer is that the student in a lecture is usually passive and sometimes asleep—a condition not conducive to maximum learning."

There are five techniques that we recommend to teachers to maintain attention: questioning, brainstorming, demonstration, role playing, and problem solving.

Questioning

In their studies of college teaching, Ellner and Barnes (1983) came to three major conclusions. First, teachers talk a lot. In typical classes, professors talked 70% of the time even in those classes that were not large lecture classes. Second, teachers spent very little time asking questions—as little as 4% of the time. Third, one-third of the questions were never answered by students, partly as the result of the fact that most questions were low level and answered by the teacher when students did not answer immediately.

Studies of questioning show that most teachers are unwilling to wait for an answer. Rowe (1974), the leading investigator in this field, has found mean "wait times" of 1.2 seconds in elementary schools and 1.8 seconds in high schools and colleges. To our knowledge, medical school "wait times" have not been studied, but based on personal experience, the average probably is between 1 and 3 seconds. Our goal is to encourage medical teachers to ask the audience questions that are not only factual or low level but to tolerate 5–10 seconds of silence before rephrasing the question and giving the answer. Since the intent of the questioning technique in a lecture is to reengage the listeners thinking, teachers should use "open" rather than "closed" questions. Open-ended questions ask for the use of information, and more than one answer may be acceptable. Close-ended questions ask for information recall and are not as stimulating. For example, asking, "Why might irritation to the diaphram result in shoulder pain?" would stimulate more thinking than, "Which nerve carries pain signals from the diaphram?"

In addition to asking questions, teachers should consider accepting questions from learners. Traditionally, this is done at the end of medical lectures. However, an effective teaching technique is to ask 20 minutes into a lecture, "I have been presenting information that is new for most of you. At this point, do you have any questions about the material we have covered?" These questions can lead to important clarification and help set the agenda for the rest of the lecture. Allowing listeners to ask questions gives them some control of the educational experience and can help wandering minds refocus on the subject at hand.

When audience members ask questions, it is important for the teacher to repeat each question so that everyone in the audience can hear the question. Also, an effective way to maintain attention is to welcome other audience members to answer the questions.

Brainstorming

Brainstorming is a special type of questioning in which the teacher asks an open-ended question and welcomes as many responses as possible. Its basic ground rule is that all answers are acceptable (although not necessarily correct). By suspending judgment on the responses, the teacher is encouraging the audience to be freewheeling and inventive. This is an excellent technique for maintaining attention on the subject.

When using the technique of brainstorming, the responses should be written on a flip chart or blackboard. To make it easier for the teacher to elicit responses and call on students, it might be helpful to ask an audience member to be the recorder. After all responses have been recorded, the teacher then might comment on their appropriateness.

As an example, in a lecture on "how to lecture," a good brainstorming question would be, "Thinking about the best lecture you have ever heard, what made it so?" After generating and recording as many responses as possible, the teacher could make comments and perhaps organize the responses into categories, e.g., process versus content. As was the case with questioning, the results of a brainstorming technique could be used to direct the next phase of the lecture, again giving the learners some control over their educational experience.

Demonstrating

Many medical lecturers use the demonstration technique quite effectively. We strongly recommend it when an experiment or actual performance will illustrate an important principle or show how something is done. Its main advantage is that it can bridge the gap between theory and practice. When well executed, a demonstration can provide an audience with a memorable experience.

Unfortunately, when demonstrations do not work, they lose rather than hold attention. Thus, it is important to practice and rehearse the demonstration so that it will work in class. Teachers need to take into account the size of the room and the audience because students who cannot see the demonstration will lose attention.

Medical lecturers have the advantage of being able to present a live patient in their demonstrations. For instance, in the chronic pain lecture that was used as an earlier example in this chapter, that lecturer could have interviewed a patient with chronic low back pain to demonstrate the involvement of cognitive and emotional factors. Using a patient in a demonstration is memorable and meaningful to medical students, residents, and other clinicians; it certainly maintains audience attention.

Role Playing

Role playing is like a demonstration, except that it requires participation by audience members. In role playing, a person adopts an assigned role and behaves in ways characteristic of that person in a specific situation. Role playing can be an effective lecture technique. For example, in a lecture on chronic pain role playing could be used to portray doctor-patient interactions: A resident takes the history of another resident who plays the role of the patient. When using this technique, it is important to be as specific as possible in assigning roles and in describing the situation in which the roles are to be played. Often, it is helpful to give written directions to each player that can be studied for 1 or 2 minutes before the role play.

When planning a role play to maintain attention, perhaps midlecture, teachers should predetermine how long they will allow for the role play. Once the role play starts, teachers should avoid interrupting until they are through with it. Then, time should be allowed for discussion, with comments by the role players. Also, audience members should be asked for their observations. Thus, the role-playing technique may require a total of 15 minutes, 5 minutes for the actual role play and 10 minutes for debriefing. Because of the time required, medical teachers might consider using this technique to maintain attention in long lectures, for example those scheduled for 1½ hours rather than only 1 hour.

Problem Solving

Problem solving is an activity that leads to the best but not necessarily the sole answer (Woods et al. 1979). Clinicians have long wondered whether they can teach medical students and residents to be better problem solvers. In a study of medical problem solving conducted by Elstein and associates (1978), it was found that better diagnosticians did not solve medical problems differently from weaker problem solvers. The differences were found in the repertory of their clinical experiences stored in long-term memory. Better diagnosticians were able to see more connections to past clinical experiences and to detect patterns. These findings in medical problem solving were confirmed in subsequent studies in the field of physics, in which expert scientists demonstrated the ability to evoke particular information to a problem at hand more rapidly than others (Larkin et al. 1980).

In one sense, these results are disappointing. If the barrier to becoming a better medical problem solver were learning the "right" steps, all that medical educators would have to do would be to teach those steps to medical students and reinforce these in residents. However, the right steps seem to be there already, genetically wired. Instead, what is needed to become better medical problem solvers is a repertory of medical problems to solve. Thus, using problems in a lecture ultimately will help make learners better problem solvers as well as maintain their attention in a lecture. At the least, information learned in the context of a problem is better remembered and used in the future (Whitman 1983).

Depending upon the time available and size of a class, audience members can be asked to solve a medical problem alone or in a small group. For example, a lecturer could provide relevant parts of a patient's data base and ask for a diagnosis and/or treatment plan.

Although it occurs to many medical teachers to use patient cases as problems, research studies also can be used as problems. For example, the lecturer could describe briefly the methodology of a published research study and ask the audience members to hypothesize the results. Then, the actual results can be presented and discussed.

We would like to present a medical education research study for two reasons. First, it provides a good example of how a research study can be used as a problem-solving technique to maintain attention in a lecture, and, second, the results of the study have great significance for physician teachers. For the sake of this example, readers should imagine themselves attending a 90-minute lecture on "How to Give a Lecture." The lecturer has attracted attention, perhaps with an anecdote about teaching. Information about lecturing has been presented for 20 minutes. To help maintain attention, the speaker uses the technique of problem solving, saying the following:

> In a study conducted by Naftulin and associates (1973), a professional actor was instructed to teach charismatically, but nonsubstantively, on a topic about which he knew nothing, "Mathematical Game Theory as Applied to Physician Education." The actor, introduced as "Dr. Myron L. Fox," was introduced with a fictitious curriculum vitae. Basically, he was trained to say nothing, but to say it beautifully. According to the audience that attended the live lecture as well as those who viewed it on videotape, Dr. Fox used enough ex-

amples to clarify his materials, presented his material in a well-organized form, and stimulated their thinking. One audience member even claimed to have read the speaker's publications. No one detected the lecture for the charade that it was!

In a follow-up study, Ware and Williams (1975) argued that the authors in the original Dr. Fox study went too far in claiming that participants had been seduced into thinking that they had learned. They pointed out that, in the first study, subjects were not asked to rate the learning gain and no measure of learning achievement was used. To improve upon the earlier study, Ware and Williams hired the same actor and instructed him to lecture to medical students on the biochemistry of memory. The students were randomly assigned to six groups. The actor delivered a high-content lecture (26 teaching points), a medium-content lecture (14 teaching points), and a low-content lecture (4 teaching points). Each level of content was presented with either high or low seduction. High-seduction behaviors included enthusiasm, humor, friendliness, expressiveness, and charisma. The researchers administered to the students an achievement test which tested the 26 items presented in the high-content lecture. In Figure 5.1, a 2 x 3 matrix shows the six lectures. Place a 1 in the box for the student group which you think did best on the achievement test. Then rank the remaining groups, 2 through 6, using a 6 for the group that did worst.

The reader should imagine that after the audience members hypothesize the results, the speaker could conduct a short discussion, comparing hypothesized with actual results. The actual results are shown in Figure 5.2.

We find it noteworthy that the low content–high seduction group tied the high content–low seduction group. In other words, students retained as much information when less information was given effec-

	High content	Medium content	Low content
High seduction	?	?	?
Low seduction	?	?	?

FIG. 5.1 Hypothesized student achievement following Dr. Fox's lecture.

	High content	Medium content	Low content
High seduction	1	2	3–4
Low seduction	3–4	5	6

FIG. 5.2 Actual student achievement following Dr. Fox's lecture.

tively as when more information was given ineffectively! This study reinforces our view that effective lecturing depends upon an interaction between process and content.

Questioning, brainstorming, demonstration, role playing, and problem solving constitute the teacher's armamentarium, the doctor's black bag. These techniques are available to the lecturer for maintaining audience attention. Having used the Dr. Fox study as an example of the problem-solving technique, we would like to address the issue it raised, i.e., content versus process.

Teaching Tips

Good content is essential to an effective lecture. It is important that the lecturer present new information that is correct, up-to-date, and relevant to the needs of learners. We have also emphasized the importance of making the material memorable and meaningful. At this time, we want to address *how* to present information effectively. There are a number of teaching tips that can be learned and practiced that will increase the effectiveness of a lecture and that apply to all public speaking situations.

The major principle of good public speaking is to be conversational. This means emphatically that teachers should not read their presentation to the audience. Speakers should deliver their lectures as if they were telling a story to one person. An outline or sketchy notes can be helpful. However, our experience is that teachers who bring a script of their presentation for "reference" purposes find themselves reading it. Using natural hand gestures and looking at listeners, one at a time with direct eye contact, is recommended. Speaking too slowly or too quickly is to be avoided, and lecturers should vary the pitch and force of their speech as they do in normal conversation.

The downfall for some speakers is the distracting mannerism, e.g., constantly clearing one's voice, saying "ah" between words, or jiggling a piece of chalk. The first (and often last) step in breaking one of these bad habits is to be aware of it. Many lecturers are not. We suggest that teachers invite a close colleague for the sole purpose of identifying distracting mannerisms. Also, having a videotape of a lecture can help identify whether any mannerisms are distracting.

If there is a distracting mannerism, then a cognitive and behavioral approach can be used to correct it:

1. Mentally rehearse an upcoming lecture and imagine making the presentation without the undesirable behaviors. Athletes have found this approach helpful in the improvement of their performances, and it is one of the basic principles of sports psychology.
2. Create a mental image to help eliminate a behavior. For example, if a teacher plays with his hair, he could imagine 5-lb weights sewn into his shirt cuffs, helping to keep his hands from reaching for his hair.
3. Write on the lecture outline or notes, "I will not . . ." and look at that statement during the presentation as a reminder.
4. Ask a colleague to observe the lecture and monitor progress or repeat the videotape process. Teachers should anticipate gradual improvement rather than extinction of a mannerism in one lecture.

Mental rehearsal is valuable for more than removing distracting mannerisms. It is helpful to practice lectures, both mentally and actually, to routinize the lecture. This does not mean memorization. It does mean becoming confident of what is to be said and done next in a lecture. Some teachers say they are more effective when they are spontaneous. Ironically, making a lecture more routine will result in more spontaneity. Speakers who are more sure of the lecture material will feel more free to alter their plans and respond to unexpected situations.

When a speaker has to think about what to say and do next, it is difficult to be spontaneous. A personal anecdote might be helpful here. When one of the authors (N.W.) was not yet an experienced lecturer, he was giving a lecture which was not routinized to a class of dental students. Each step of the way, he was concerned about his next words. The lecture seemed to be going well, except for one problem. Periodically, the class laughed in unison. There was a joke that everyone was getting except him. He checked, and his fly was not open. He was wondering, "What is so funny?" Finally, a colleague handed him a note. The teacher was referring repeatedly to a study by "Sherlock and Holmes," when the actual authors were Sherlock and Morris!

In addition to rehearsal, preparing a class handout can help routinize a lecture, particularly when the handout includes the instructional objectives, an outline, key points, and references. Earlier in this chapter, we discussed why presenting a lecture potentially is more effective than handing out a text of the lecture for students to read on their own. Medical teachers often ask what they should hand out to students. Students differ in their ability to take notes, and a complete text would provide all learners with an accurate record of the lecture. However, this type of handout encourages passivity. Students may not attend class if they could obtain the text, and those in class may not actively listen.

Providing only a skeletal handout would encourage active listening, but some students have difficulty taking notes and listening. Russell and colleagues (1983) studied the effect of giving medical students a comprehensive manuscript of the lecture containing text and tables, a partial handout that included key points and illustrations, and a skeleton outline. In general, they found that students preferred the comprehensive manuscript, but that students with partial or skeletal handouts performed better on written examinations. They concluded that the partial handout was the best compromise between a complete manuscript that encourages passivity and a skeletal handout that encourages alertness in class but may be less valuable for later review.

We conclude this chapter with some specific comments about a special type of lecture, grand rounds. Some physicians feel that grand rounds no longer live up to the standards of the past (Ingelfinger 1972). Late in the 19th century, attending physicians conducted grand rounds by walking through the wards and stopping at the bedside of interesting patients. When the trail of white coats (the proverbial "mass of shifting dullness") became too large for the wards, grand rounds were shifted to the hospital's auditorium, but the use of patients was preserved. Today, however, few grand rounds incorporate a live patient. Although a patient case may be presented, the grand rounds is otherwise indistinguishable from other lectures.

We would like to see more grand rounds address specific patient problems that highlight the interconnectedness of social, economic, psychological, and physical problems, the biopsychosocial approach advocated by Engel (1965). We encourage physician teachers to elicit audience participation, welcoming their questions and asking for their comments on the case. It can be productive to withhold until late in the presentation results that will reveal the final diagnosis and treatment plan. We would like to see teachers keep in mind that grand rounds should be more than a topical lecture . . . it should be a problem-oriented exercise (for the audience).

Conclusion

We recognize that there is too much lecturing in medical school and that too many lectures are boring. Lectures can be stimulating if information not easily found in print is presented. In particular, lecturers should aim to convey new knowledge as well as an understanding of it. Presenters can attract attention with an anecdote, story, or question, as well as a statement of purpose, maintain attention with techniques such as questioning, brainstorming, demonstration, role playing, or problem-solving exercise. There *is* a relationship between content and process: Good speaking skills *do* make a difference.

CHAPTER 6

Group Discussions

It is said that Woodrow Wilson, when teaching at Princeton, would stride into his classroom, greet the class, and then say, "Gentlemen, are there any questions?" If no questions were asked then the class would be dismissed, since it was Professor Wilson's contention that his young scholars had not prepared for class that day (Braughman 1974, p. 126).

In chapter 5, we suggested how to improve medical lectures. Once teachers have achieved this goal, we suggest that they give fewer lectures. We support the recommendation of the GPEP report (Association of American Medical Colleges 1984) that alternative methods be used to achieve more than the transfer of information. While suggesting fewer lectures and more group discussions, we acknowledge the difficulties posed for the teacher. As dramatized by the story about Woodrow Wilson, leading group discussion requires the teacher to depend on the preparation of the students. Compared to lecturing, leading group discussions requires that the teacher and the learners share responsibility for the instructional process. As explained by one award-winning teacher, "Because discussion is much more unpredictable than lecturing, it requires considerable instructor spontaneity, creativity, and tolerance for the unknown (Lowman 1984, p. 119). Although difficult to master, group discussion can be rewarding for teachers and learners when used properly and for the appropriate objectives.

Objectives

In the last chapters, we suggested that all lectures should address one general affective objective: "This subject is worth knowing." However, more specific affective objectives can be addressed in group discussions, e.g., "chronic pain should not be confused with symptom faking and malingering." Whenever a teacher wants to influence feelings, values, or attitudes, change will occur only if learners are actively involved. This active role is provided for by group discussion. In a group discussion, all participants have the opportunity to express their own views and to hear those of others; positions on issues can be challenged, and different views can be incorporated into new positions.

When an existing attitude might interfere with achieving cognitive objectives, then a group discussion should precede a lecture. For example, a medical teacher might wish to lecture on the treatment of alcoholism. However, medical students might believe that treatment of alcoholic patients is a waste of time. Unless the affective objective of "believing that the treatment of alcoholic patients is worthwhile" is achieved first, then the lecture would be a waste of time.

In addition to addressing affective objectives, group discussions are suitable for achieving higher-level cognitive objectives. In the last chapter, we suggested that lower-level cognitive objectives, i.e., knowledge and comprehension, can be achieved in lectures, but that achievement of application objectives requires an opportunity to use the information in new situations, which is possible in group discussions. Moreover, the active student role allowed by a group discussion provides teachers with an opportunity to observe and assess the learners engaged in the application process. Also, the higher cognitive objectives of analysis, synthesis, and evaluation definitely require the active role allowed by group discussions.

When learners have not yet achieved the lower cognitive objectives, then the higher cognitive objectives cannot be achieved, even in a group discussion. When group discussion leaders try to engage learners in analysis, synthesis, or evaluation of material not well known or understood by them, participation becomes forced and unmeaningful. For example, if medical students do not know or understand the treatment modalities of alcoholism, then they cannot be expected to discuss a patient case and evaluate his treatment. Thus, a lecture should precede the group discussion to provide knowledge and comprehension.

Leading group discussions requires preparation and facilitative skills. According to one teacher, "As is painfully apparent to well-meaning instructors who have tried to stimulate classroom discussions by simply showing up, successful and exciting sessions do not just happen" (Barnes-McConnell 1980, p. 62).

Techniques

Questioning is the major technique used to "make discussion happen." In the last chapter on lecturing, we suggested that open questions were more stimulating than closed questions. In group discussions, closed questions can be helpful to assess the knowledge level of participants and to start discussion. However, prolonged use of close questions turns a group discussion into an oral quiz. Thus, it is particularly important for group discussion leaders to develop the skill of formulating open-ended questions that will stimulate discussion. These questions are similar to those used in taking the history of a patient. For group discussion purposes, we recommend a repertoire of four types of open-ended questions: broadening, justifying, hypothetical, and alternative.

Broadening questions ask participants to go beyond the stated facts. For example, in a group discussion of abdominal pain, a teacher might present the case of a 43-year-old man who arrives at the emergency room at 6:00 AM, complaining of abdominal pain (Pestana 1985). He is lying on the stretcher on his back, with his knees drawn up. The man changes position, lying on his side, but still with his knees drawn up and vomits a small amount of greenish fluid. A broadening question would be, "The fact that the patient sought help at an inconvenient hour suggests that the pain is severe. What other clues are important?" One possible response would be that the fetal position suggests pancreatic pain. Another student might comment that perforated ulcer was a possibility. The teacher could then ask, "How well does the presence of greenish fluid match up with that diagnosis?"

Justifying questions are used to challenge old ideas and develop new ones. For example, the teacher might continue: "The man was in good health until he returned at 8:00 PM from a party at which he ate and drank heavily. The pain began gradually and built up to a high level of intensity in half an hour. The pain was severe, constant, and radiated to the back. What diagnoses do you have in mind now?" A discussant might suggest alcoholic gastritis. The teacher could ask, "Why do you think so?" After the student's defense of this diagnosis, the group discussion leader could ask others if they agree. It is better for someone else rather than the teacher to suggest that alcoholic gastritis might have been partially relieved with vomiting and likely would have produced bleeding. However, a group discussion should not become a "guessing game," and the discussion leader should be willing to provide information not known to other participants.

Hypothetical questions are used to change the course of discussion. For example, if the patient had a serum amylase of 180, the teacher could ask, "How would the significance of this finding change if the abdominal pain had been present 48 instead of 10 hours?" The points made in discussion might include that elevation of serum amylase usually occurs early in the disease and disappears early, in about 1 or 2 days.

Alternative questions are used to develop options. In this case, the teacher could ask, "If an elevated serum amylase is seen in 48 hours, what additional test would you consider?" A discussant might suggest a urine amylase test. The teacher then could ask, "If that were elevated, what would be your next step?" One response could be an abdominal CAT scan.

By using broadening, justifying, hypothetical, and alternative questions, group discussion leaders provide opportunities for learners to apply, analyze, synthesize, and evaluate their knowledge. If students cannot answer these types of questions, then the group discussion leader can conclude that the students have not yet achieved the knowledge and comprehension objectives that are a prerequisite for the achievement of the higher-level objectives.

In the last chapter, we described brainstorming as a special type of questioning that can be used to maintain attention in a lecture. Brainstorming also is useful in group discussions, especially to help a group solve problems. According to Osborne (1963), the originator of brainstorming, creative problem solving consists of finding facts, ideas, and solutions. Brainstorming is a good technique to help a group find facts, ideas, and solutions. It is particularly helpful when a problem lends itself to many solutions, for example, generating a diagnosis for a patient presenting with abdominal pain. When using brainstorming, group discussion leaders should orient participants to its ground rules:

1. _Criticism is ruled out._ The group discussion leader should defer judgment and direct other group members to do the same.
2. _Freewheeling is welcomed._ The group discussion leader should give positive reinforcement to all contributions.
3. _Quantity is wanted._ The more ideas, the better.
4. _Combination is encouraged._ The group discussion leader should motivate participants to build on each others ideas.

Questioning and brainstorming are the major techniques of group discussion leaders. At times, the learners may challenge this format. For example, suppose one medical student says, "I don't understand where this discussion is going. Why don't you just tell us what you want us to know?" A teacher who was uncommitted to the group discussion process might respond, "I'm glad you asked. Here's what I think you need to know." The discussion ends and everyone listens attentively. A defensive teacher might respond, "I want you to think for yourselves. What good would it do if I gave you answers all the time?" The other students would then be reluctant to share their thoughts and feelings.

A more constructive approach would be to acknowledge the student's need for direction by responding, "I can see that the discussion may have lost its direction for you. Can you summarize what we have covered so far and see if you can help us get on track?" Perhaps, an even more facilitative approach would be to involve the whole group by responding, "I have a feeling others may feel the same way. Perhaps, before we continue, we should summarize what we have covered so far. Would someone begin by suggesting some of the points?"

The principle we wish to impart here is that successful group discussion leadership requires a strong, but not defensive, commitment to the process. While leaders are responsible for establishing a supportive environment, they should engage all participants in solving the group's problems if any occur.

Tips

During the 1930s, when discussion groups became fashionable, the U.S. Department of Agriculture sent a teacher throughout the country to show farmers how to participate in meetings (Zander 1979). The teacher, Drummond Jones, would begin a day-long session by asking participants what properties could prevent discussions from being effective and then ask them to consider these causes. Halfway through the day, he would ask them to comment on how he had helped or hindered their discussion. Their comments helped identify the leadership procedures that improved the quality of a meeting.

These leadership procedures are different from lecture skills. In fact, some physician teachers whose repertoire of facts and entertaining delivery style have led to great success as lecturers fail miserably as group discussion leaders. Several authors have described in general terms the teacher behaviors associated with successful group discussion leadership (Rubeck & Pratt 1979; Foley & Smilansky 1980; Barnes-McConnell 1980). To these we have added our personal experience and propose three basic areas of behavior and attitude that are important to effective group leadership (Whitman & Schwenk 1983):

Comfortable With Dialogue and Interpersonal Interaction

Not all teachers are comfortable with group discussion as a teaching modality, perhaps, because there is a loss of control by the teacher. When the communication is not largely one way, the instructor must accept the notion that all who participate share the leadership of the teaching process as well as responsibility for its success or failure.

The sharing of leadership and responsibility is made clear when the group discussion leader sets ground rules for the discussion, such as, "I will not be lecturing to you today. Your questions and views are not only acceptable, but essential, to the learning that will take place." By being explicit, the group discussion leader can set into motion an interactive process. However, as Brookfield (1985, p. 63) has pointed out, "Discussions do not exhibit intellectual elegance and equity of participation simply because a teacher has decreed that a group is to engage in a discussion." Thus, crucial to the success of a group discussion is agreement by participants of common purposes and behaviors.

While teachers give up a degree of control in group discussion, compared to lectures, they do not give up all control. The degree to which control is shared varies considerably. Some groups should be "learner centered." For example, suppose that the topic of congestive heart failure is to be addressed by a group of residents. If the purpose is to decide if a patient was managed properly, then the attending physician might allow participants to take responsibility for the outcome of the discussion. However, if the participants were third-year medical students, then the same discussion leader might choose a more "teacher centered" approach, directing questions to students and providing information as needed. Moreover, some discussions should be "group centered," with teacher and students participating equally. For example, an attending physician, residents, and students might discuss the ethical issues raised in the management of a congestive heart failure patient.

Capacity for Professional Intimacy

In a manner analogous to doctor-patient relationships, teachers should be close to students without necessarily becoming personal friends. Being "professionally" intimate implies an ability and willingness to reveal personal thoughts and feelings relevant to the teaching-learning process. For example, an attending should be willing to express discomfort with how the congestive heart failure patient was managed. By sharing personal views, the group discussion leader is encouraging others to do the same.

Teachers who are professionally intimate bring authenticity to the teacher-student relationship. By being honest and open with their learners, teachers can see themselves as members of a joint partnership with learners, learning from each other. This will help prevent an adversarial relationship from developing. For example, the clinician's willingness to say "I don't know." will discourage others from playing the "pretend to know" game that unfortunately characterizes many group discussions.

The pretend-to-know game is highlighted in the story (Black 1985) about the attending physician who asks a group of medical students, "What is the true function of the spleen?" One student, thinking he is supposed to know it, says, "I forgot." Of course, forgetting sounds better then never having known. To this, the attending replies, "What a shame. The one person in the world who knows, and he forgot." The penalty we pay for the playing of this game often is missed learning opportunities.

Ability to Create a Tension Level That Enhances Learning

Less learning occurs when there is too little or too much stress; more learning occurs when there is an optimal stress that challenges without threatening (Whitman et al. 1984). Group leaders can create an appropriate tension level when they ask questions that push the thinking of participants. Also, it is important to use questions that will involve all members of the group.

Another key to optimizing the stress level is nonjudgmental acceptance of student statements without implying agreement with every statement. For example, if a student is simply wrong about a medical fact, the leader should correct it or ask another participant to do so. As was pointed out in a survey of third- and fourth-year medical students, it is important to correct students without belittling them (Stritter et al. 1975).

Disagreement over an opinion can be more difficult. In this case, the discussion leader might say, "I understand what you are saying, but I'm not sure I agree. I wonder what others think." At some point, the discussion leader should offer a personal opinion. This may be necessary to be professionally intimate. The key is to do so without overwhelming the students with teacher opinions.

Kenneth Eble (1979, p. 60), former director of the Project to Improve College Teaching, sponsored by the American Association of University Professors and the American Association of Colleges, has emphasized the importance of being ingeniously responsive to students' answers and questions: "No utterances are wrong; though they may be false . . . never deliberately ignore a question or demean the questioner."

By being comfortable with interpersonal interaction, being professionally intimate, and creating an optimal tension and stress level, group discussion leaders can aim for a rhythm in a sequence of questions and answers that leads a group to achieving "moments of greater understanding" (Eble 1979, p. 68). Clinicians aim at a similar rhythm in their dialogues with patients.

To achieve a rhythm that is energetic without being hectic, discussion leaders should learn to tolerate silence after asking a question. However, many teachers are uncomfortable with silence and answer their own questions. When directing a question to an individual, we recommend waiting at least 3 seconds before rephrasing or calling on someone else. When asking the whole group, at least 5 seconds is recommended. These "wait times" seem short, but in actual practice, many group discussion leaders wait only for 1 or 2 seconds (Rowe 1974). Also, when a question has been answered, teachers should wait 1 or 2 seconds before giving feedback. This allows the respondent to add more and also allows other participants to evaluate the answer.

Conclusion

We recognize that there is a need to increase the use of group discussion. However, many medical teachers may feel uncomfortable with the degree of control that is lost when leading discussions rather than delivering lectures. Nevertheless, group discussions are essential if addressing attitudes and achieving higher-level cognitive objectives are to occur. We suggest that through the use of questioning, teachers can share with their learners responsibility for the teaching-learning interaction, establish a personal yet professional rapport with learners, and create a tension level that challenges everyone's best thinking.

CHAPTER 7

Teaching Rounds and Morning Report

The task faced by the clinical teacher "is unique in the entire realm of teaching. In no other field does the nature of the material demand of the teacher this degree of preparedness without preparation." (Reichsman et al. 1964 in Mattern et al. 1983)

The authors have experienced (unfortunately more than once) teaching rounds and morning reports like the following instances:

1. The attending is well known for arriving late and leaving early for morning report, because of his own research and clinical demands. Knowing this, the admitting resident presents the most complicated patient admission first. As the resident finishes his presentation, the attending (who has arrived in the middle of the morning report) makes a few superficial remarks and abruptly leaves rounds to the supervision of the chief resident, who takes the team off to do the morning's work.

2. During the course of the case presentation, practically every resident is paged to the telephone for at least part of the presentation, so that by the end no one is able to discuss the entire case. The larger group discussion deteriorates to a two-party discussion of treatment plans by the attending physician and the admitting resident, with the

rest of the ward team looking bored and wanting to get on to their ward work.

3. After the case presentation is finished, a senior resident makes a number of clinically provocative statements about a relatively minor aspect of the case. Another resident rises to the challenge, causing an argument that the other residents neither understand nor appreciate. They leave the conference room one by one as they are paged.

4. A complex patient is presented and the attending and the chief resident enter into an important discussion about how to best handle an anticipated complication, a discussion that is not understood at all by any of the students or interns. The plan is determined. As the team prepares to see the patient to initiate the plan, the attending asks the students if they have any questions. They all shake their heads, "No."

As is common in medical education, there are often strong conflicts in teaching rounds between patient care needs and educational objectives. Often, the balance seems to frequently weigh too heavily toward service needs, to the detriment of educational needs. The purpose of this chapter is to provide teaching techniques and tips to help the attending physician accomplish the "work" of work rounds, teaching rounds, and morning report comfortably, and simultaneously, with the educational work. While the intern is struggling to understand the most serious diagnoses a patient might have, the chief resident is teaching brainstorming and deductive reasoning. While the residents are anxiously working to understand the physiology of a complex ICU patient, the attending physician is demonstrating the ability to critique and modify previous treatment decisions, thereby modeling the behaviors of a mature and seasoned clinician. The activities and outcomes of day-to-day patient care not only can, but must, coexist peacefully with the teaching of clinical problem solving and decision making.

Objectives

Every teacher-learner interaction has learning objectives. According to Bloom and colleagues' (1956) taxonomy of objectives, higher-order cognitive objectives and affective objectives are best accomplished with tutorial and group discussion formats, of which teaching rounds and morning report are examples. These higher order objectives include *analysis, synthesis, evaluation,* and *changes in professional demeanor* and *affect.* The types of skills that are best learned in this format are *independent reasoning* and *clinical judgment, effective communication of clinical material,* and the *art of critique and clinical consultation.* While teaching rounds may not be the most appropriate format for transmitting certain facts about the anatomy of the peritoneal cavity (see chapter 5, Lectures), it is perhaps the only way of effectively teaching how to evaluate and manage a patient with abdominal pain. To meet these learning objectives, the teacher has five teaching strategies, which are discussed next.

Establish an Efficient Format That Satisfies Time Constraints

The easiest way to fail in meeting the educational objectives of teaching rounds is to take so long in doing so that the admitting residents mentally (or physically) leave rounds in order to get their daily work done. Contrary to popular thinking in medical education, more is rarely better. An efficient and succinct approach to each patient in which important, but not necessarily all, points are highlighted is clearly the most productive for both patient care and learning. An efficient format balances the conflicting time needs of patient care (less time) and teaching (more time), and balances the conflicting time needs of students (more time), residents (less time), and attending physicians (usually less depending on other demands). Most new patients can be adequately (not necessarily completely) discussed in 10 or 15 minutes, although complex patients may take as much as 20 or 30 minutes. Previously admitted patients should require much less time, unless significant complications require the initiation of a major new discussion.

Teach Simultaneously at Several Levels of Learner Experience and Knowledge

Teaching rounds are not lectures. An important goal of teaching rounds is to teach the process of clinical decision making and problem solving. In order for this learning to occur, it seems logical that students and residents of all levels of experience need to do a little work: to venture guesses and opinions, to ask questions, and to challenge others. These things will not happen if only one or two participants do all the talking. The role of the attending physician is to guarantee equal access to "air time" for all concerned. All opinions are not equally brilliant or helpful to the patient care process—the most efficient group for providing care is a group of one. However, all opinions can become vehicles for learning by those who hold them, propose them, receive the appropriate feedback, and revise them. This process is absolutely critical to successful learning and cannot be avoided or short-circuited.

Promote Clinical Problem Solving as the Goal of Teaching Rounds

The ultimate goal of teaching rounds and morning report is to teach the art of clinical problem solving and decision making at the same time that actual problems are being solved and actual decisions are being made. The role of the experienced attending physician is crucial to the achievement of this combined educational and patient care goal. Most helpful will be the ability to make the clinical reasoning process visible, apparent and explicit, rather than hidden, mystical, and inexplicable, as it often appears to students.

Clinical decision making is a deductive process in which empirically tested paradigms directly link hypotheses to a physical examination finding, laboratory result, historical information. The experience of the attending physician must be made apparent in this process. Clinical problem solving has long been thought to be a higher-order cognitive process, the steps for which could be listed, taught, and learned. Researchers searched for the "magical" list of steps. The list was delineated, but, to the surprise of many, the same list was used by both experienced and inexperienced physicians (Whitman 1983; Elstein et al. 1978). This was disappointing to many educators who had hoped that teaching clinical problem solving could be accomplished by simply teaching the set of steps previously unknown to the student and inexperienced resident. Instead, clinical problem solving, as a learning objective, is a skill with steps that can be easily demonstrated but require extensive and continued practice. "The difference between experts and weaker problem solvers [is found more] in the repertoire of their experiences, organized in long-term memory, than in differences in the planning and problem-solving heuristics employed" (Elstein et al. 1978, p. 276). What this means for attending physicians is that _every patient presentation and every patient care encounter with a student must be turned into an opportunity for explicit demonstration and guided practice in clinical problem solving._ This goal should guide the teacher in all teaching rounds and morning report activities.

Provide Feedback and Personal Evaluations to Learners

In a well-described seminar method for improving the clinical teaching of attending physicians, Skeff and associates (1984) list the provision of constructive feedback and personal evaluations at the end of a rotation as one of the critical skills to be mastered by clinical teachers. Mattern and associates (1983) noted that while attending physicians were somewhat uncomfortable in providing face-to-face evaluations to learners, the learners felt this information had significant educational value and correlated well with the overall value of the educational experience. These authors (Mattern et al. 1983, p. 1130) also noted "that constructive criticism could be offered frankly and tactfully, without compromising the role of the attending physician as a mentor, potential friend, or future advocate. Such conversations often served as a bridge extending the relationship of the learners to the attending physician beyond the brief lifetime of the group." While the distinction between evaluation that is *formative* (used to improve future performance) and *summative* (used to assess past performance) is critical (see chapter 4), the need for attending physicians to provide more of both is even more so. Many studies confirm the desire of learners to receive more feedback about their performance (Gil et al. 1984), although experienced teachers suspect that the learners really want to hear more positive feedback in particular. In any case, the importance of providing feedback and summative evaluation cannot be overemphasized. Summative evaluation, in particular, "must be given the attention that it requires, because the material that accrues in a trainee's folder becomes the basis on which recommendations for further education, certification, employment, or remedial work must be made" (Reuler et al. 1980, p. 236).

Bring Closure to Both Patient Care Issues and the Teaching Process

Since teaching rounds have both patient care and educational objectives, the accomplishment of one without the other is a hollow victory. Patient presentations that close only with diagnostic and treatment plans passed gratuitously from teacher to learner cheat learners out of an opportunity, never again available, to check understanding, to debate options, to critically exam the thinking of others, and to practice the skills of clinical problem solving. Patient problems that are debated forever in a divergent, open-ended fashion, as if on a television talk show, leave learners with too much instruction and too little supervision and guidance, to the detriment of patient care and the development of appropriate professional behaviors by the learner. Leaving rounds with several ideas about how to proceed does neither the patient nor the learner any good if the best one of those ideas is not selected and implemented.

Techniques

To carry out these teaching strategies and to achieve the learning objectives, teachers have available many possible techniques. Not all techniques are applicable in every situation, and some techniques are never applicable with certain teachers. While certain general characteristics of good teaching and good teachers do exist, variety and even idiosyncrasy still have their place. This disclaimer is made to allow the reader the freedom to experiment and explore without the burden of wondering if he is following the "one right way" of teaching. The teaching techniques useful in teaching rounds and morning report, which are organized into five basic areas, are presented next.

Model the General Characteristics of Good Clinical Teachers

The characteristics of excellent clinical teachers have been extensively studied (Stritter et al. 1975; Stritter & Hain 1977; Irby, 1978 Irby & Rakestraw 1981; Mattern et al. 1983; Lamkin et al. 1983), and the results of these studies are essentially identical. Some studies surveyed the characteristics of ideal teachers as perceived by learners, others as perceived by teachers, and still others as perceived by both; again, the results are remarkably similar. Both learners and teachers agreed that clinical teachers should

1. Possess an excellent fund of knowledge;
2. Explicitly demonstrate excellent clinical judgement;
3. Be adept at interacting interpersonally with students and residents;
4. Show enthusiasm for the teaching role itself.

Students on an obstetrics and gynecology rotation described four factors that contribute to overall teacher effectiveness (Irby & Rakestraw 1981):

1. Good supervisory skills, including providing appropriate direction and feedback to students, actively involving students in clinical activities and being accessible to student questions and needs;
2. Excellent knowledge, including being clear, analytical and organized in presentations and discussions;
3. Good interpersonal relationships, including establishing rapport and being enthusiastic and stimulating;
4. Clinical competence, including demonstrating good skills, procedures, and patient care abilities.

In an earlier hallmark study (Stritter et al. 1975), all third- and fourth-year students at a medical school were surveyed regarding the characteristics of the ideal clinical teacher. Of 77 possibly helpful teaching behaviors offered, the students rated 16 to be particularly successful, including approaching teaching with enthusiasm, correcting students without belittling, emphasizing conceptual comprehension over mere factual recall, preparing well for teaching rounds and patient discussions, and identifying and summarizing major and important discussion points. These 16 behaviors were further organized by factor analysis into six major factors characterizing good clinical teaching:

1. Active student participation, including providing adequate time for student-directed discussion, answering questions precisely, and remaining willingly accessible;
2. Enthusiastic attitude toward teaching, including conveying enjoyment in associating with students, demonstrating sensitivity to patient and student needs simultaneously, and demonstrating genuine interest in students through a friendly manner;
3. Emphasizing problem solving through stressing the broad applicability of knowledge, giving every student chances to practice skills and procedures, and requiring students to demonstrate thinking processes rather than merely rewarding correct answers;
4. Defining a student-centered style of instruction, including setting realistic objectives for the particular group of students concerned, assessing the progress of each student individually, demonstrating sensitivity to student concerns such as feelings of inadequacy, and giving negative and positive feedback appropriately.
5. Having a humanistic orientation, including stressing the social and psychological aspects of patient care, dealing with students and hospital personnel in a friendly, sensitive manner, and advising students on nonmedical issues when requested and appropriate;
6. Emphasizing references and appropriate research, including citing important references, challenging opinions in journals, and incorporating personal research when appropriate.

All these characteristics can be organized into the two components of creative clinical teaching (see Epilogue): innovation and usefulness. Most medical teachers are useful, competent, organized, well-read, well-prepared, possess appropriate clinical and research experience, and able to summarize important points—but they do not present a novel approach (pedantic bores). Most medical teachers probably fear being innovative but not useful (charlatans). The best choice for clinical teachers is to be both innovative *and* useful by being enthusiastic, stimulating, gentle, patient, genuinely interested in students, and accessible to students.

Use an Efficient Logistical Format for Case Presentations and Establish a Productive Learning Climate

An efficient format balances the conflict between the needs of patient care (which require less time) and teaching (which require more time), while giving learners sufficient physical comfort to encourage their participation. While new and complex patients may require more time than previously admitted patients, it is still the responsibility of the teacher to determine the caseload at the start of the meeting and plan accordingly. Carrying rounds into a 3- or 4-hour marathon is rarely educational, although it may represent an impressive demonstration by the teacher of pedantic fortitude. Presentation in Weed's (1968) well-known SOAP format should be required, even for those patients presented briefly in follow-up. Only pertinent positive and negative points should be included, so that even the most complicated patient can be presented in no more than 5 minutes. Yurchak (1981) notes that the "entire presentation should be completed in seven minutes. This is probably the maximum time during which a listener can give . . . his undivided attention. Beyond seven minutes, most listeners will find it impossible to retain all the facts." Complex patients do not necessarily require more time but a more careful and parsimonious selection of the data chosen for presentation. Stressing (and enforcing) this need for brevity is the responsibility of the attending.

Certain aspects of the presentation deserve emphasis. Historical information should focus almost solely on the chief complaints, with only very pertinent past history and systems review included. A modest amount of psychosocial history is important, both to give listeners a mental image of the patient as well as to provide data important for both diagnosis and treatment. Only pertinent aspects of the physical examination should be reported. The reporting of obscure signs, especially with eponyms, is to be discouraged. The reporting of laboratory findings should include a justification of costs and risks. The diagnostic assessment should include specific hypotheses in the form of a problem list and should include a defense. The clinical reasoning should be made explicit and apparent. The management plan should acknowledge acceptable alternatives. A more directed problem-solving style of case discussion is described under Technique. In whatever way the case is presented and led, the teacher is responsible for setting appropriate expectations and enforcing them, through specific feedback.

Teaching rounds have been known to occur in all types of locations, including conference rooms, hallways, cafeterias, and outdoors in good weather. Only the first location is truly conducive to focused discussion and learning. The room should have comfortable and adequate seating and allow each participant to see all others. Rounds in which the medical students stand uncomfortably in the back, or in which the entire group shuffles about as if with some vestigial memory of Oslerian days, are rarely productive. The description of these rounds as a "mass of shifting dullness" is an apt one. If bedside teaching or examination is an objective of the rotation, it is better handled at a different time, usually with a smaller group, and with defined, prearranged purposes (see chapter 8).

Finally, successful morning report and teaching rounds formats in which not all patients are ever presented or discussed do exist (Pupa & Carpenter 1985). This method, however, requires careful monitoring and documentation of the case mix and follow-up discussions, as well as an assertive approach to following selected case presentations with appropriate written materials and didactic presentations. The advantages of selecting patients for purely educational purposes are obvious, including time savings, prospective curriculum planning, and the ability to remedy undiscovered deficiencies. The disadvantage lies in the artificial nature of separating patient care from educational objectives. While it is difficult to accomplish these often conflicting purposes simultaneously, the times that are successful are remarkably helpful in modeling future self-learning behaviors for students who will have a lifetime of coexistent patient care and continuing medical educational needs.

Setting an appropriate learning climate is an instructional technique that researchers find incredibly useful but that practitioners seem to use infrequently. This discrepancy may be because "setting the learning climate" sounds too much like educational jargon, the immediate implementation of which is unclear at best. Actually, experienced attending physicians establish the learning climate almost naturally, without giving it considerable thought, by clarifying their expectations for teaching rounds; specifying the format for case presentation and discussion; creating an atmosphere that encourages open questioning and discussion; defining the way and time in which patient care issues will be brought to closure; and providing personal, constructive feedback to team members at the end of the ward rotation. Skeff et al. (1984) list setting of the learning climate as one of the critical skills developed by clinical teachers in extensive seminar and workshop experiences. This skill is manifested by establishing an appropriate tone for the teaching that is a combination of stimulation and comfort suitable to the individual teacher. Each teacher is, of course, different with regard to this tone; of importance is that the teacher's notions of appropriate stimulation and comfort be made explicit. Reuler and associates (1980) suggest holding an individual meeting with each team member to discuss the learner's past experiences, current learning objectives, and long-range goals so as to fit the teacher's expectations with those of the learner. These individual meetings can be held at the beginning of the service. Similar meetings can be held at the end of the service to provide (and receive) feedback, to make constructive criticisms, and to place the recent learning experience in the context of the learner's future assignments.

Use Divergent, Open-Ended Questioning to Promote Clinical Problem Solving

Clinical problem solving is really the ultimate learning objective of teaching rounds. Unfortunately, recent reviews (Whitman & Schwenk 1986; Elstein et al. 1978) suggest that clinical problem-solving skills may not be able to be taught directly. The skills used by excellent problem solvers are essentially the same as those of more average problem solvers. The difference between the two groups has more to do with a different repertoire of past problem-solving experiences and the ready retrievability of previously used knowledge from their long-term memories. For teachers of clinical problem solving, the most important implication of this research is that every learning activity _must_ be made into a problem-solving activity. Every learner-patient and teacher-learner interaction must be turned into a problem-solving exercise, no matter how brief. Clinical teachers can make sure that their interactions stimulate problem solving by asking questions rather than giving answers. Learners may think they are learning more by being given answers, but actually being asked questions is far more productive. The educational research clearly shows that learning increases as the learner becomes more interactive. The learner is most interactive when the teacher renews his committment to a somewhat tarnished, but now refurbished, concept of Socratic teaching. Modeling himself after Professor Kingsfield, the law school nemesis in the movie _The Paper Chase,_ may not be helpful, but a teacher's dedication to the value of questioning as the prime teaching technique in teaching rounds is highly recommended. Foley and associates (1979) have analyzed the ways in which time on teaching rounds is spent. They showed that the instructor in teaching rounds talked during 62% of the available time; students talked only 4%. The majority of that time was spent in providing information and answering questions in a relatively unstimulating and low-level fashion. This situation is to be avoided at all costs. Taylor (1984) and Skeff (1984) have shown that appropriate evaluations and teacher workshops can have a profound effect on the ability of attending physicians to adopt a more stimulating, questioning, open-ended, and nondirective style of conducting teaching rounds.

Questioning has a number of valuable educational uses in addition to its most common one, which is, of course, to ascertain whether the learner has a particular answer or fact. Faculty at the Family Practice Faculty Development Center of Texas (Lamkin et al. 1983) list, among others, the following uses:

To stimulate learning and thinking;
To assist the learner in organizing and clarifying concepts;
To correct misunderstandings or faulty reasoning (right answer but wrong reason);
To assist in showing special or obscure relationships;
To strengthen the learner's ability to synthesize and analyze;
To correct attitudes or behavior.

Mattern and associates (1983) observed that "the most successful attending strategy . . . was a composite of careful listening, limited questioning, use of clarifying rather than probing questions, and use of the student's presentation and impression as the springboard for the subsequent case discussion and analysis. . . . Use of thought-provoking questions is a powerful instructional strategy in clinical teaching, but our observations and interviews indicate that such a strategy will find its least suitable application in the middle of a case presentation." Weinholtz (1983) examined the most productive styles of questioning and types of questions more closely by studying various combinations of frequencies of questioning during the case presentation, as well as the mixture of probing versus clarifying questions used. The style and type most preferred by students was a low-frequency clarifying combination, in which questioning was infrequent and questions were benign. The combination most productive for promoting problem solving was high-frequency questioning and probing questions; this combination, which prolongs rounds, was obviously least liked by students. The best compromise between the two seems to be a medium frequency of mixed questions, beginning with clarifying questions early in the case presentation and moving to more probing questions towards the end. The difficulty for the teacher lies in gauging the number of questions to ask, how hard to probe, how to pace the questioning in the interest of efficient rounds, and how much stimulation the presenter and the team can tolerate in the face of educational anxiety and patient care demands.

Given these guidelines, we can recommend certain specific types of questions to attending physicians conducting teaching rounds and morning report. The types of questions that promote clinical problem solving are those that are open ended and divergent. Students should be asked to clarify, support, defend, justify, correlate, critique, evaluate, analyze, interpret, and predict. They should not be asked to regurgitate facts or answers with one or a few words. The following questions can be used to stimulate problem solving and critical thinking during the various stages of teaching rounds and morning report.

1. Throughout the presentation:
   "At this point in the presentation, what hypotheses do you have in mind?"
   "Why did you just ask . . . ?"
   "Explain the pathophysiology of the *[finding]* just presented."
   "What did you expect to learn from asking that question?"
   "How would what you expected to learn change your diagnosis or treatment approach?"
   "How does the information just provided change the most likely diagnosis?"
   "How does the information just provided suggest a need for immediate action?"
2. During the presentation of the history:
   "What further historical information would you like the presenter to provide?"

"Based on the historical information presented, what physical examination findings will be particularly important to note?"

"What is your evaluation of the previous medical care received by this patient?"

3. During the presentation of the physical examination:

   "What further physical examination data would you like the presenter to provide?"

   "If *[physical examination finding]* were present *[absent]* instead of absent *[present]*, how would it change your differential diagnosis?"

   "Based on the history and physical examination data presented, what laboratory tests would you recommend?"

4. During the presentation of laboratory data:

   "What further laboratory data might clarify the differential diagnosis?"

   "If *[laboratory test]* were positive *[negative]* instead of negative *[positive]*, how would it change your differential diagnosis?"

   "Justify the use of *[laboratory test]*."

   "Justify the cost of performing *[laboratory test]*."

   "What would you do if *[laboratory test]* were unavailable?"

5. During the presentation of the diagnosis and assessment:

   "What are the most likely diagnoses?"

   "What are the most serious or emergent diagnoses?"

   "What are the diagnoses that are most treatable?"

   "What pieces of information tend to support your best hypothesis?"

   "What pieces of information tend to detract from your best hypothesis?"

   "Build a case to support *[alternative hypothesis]*."

6. During the presentation of the treatment plan:

   "If *[examination finding, laboratory test, x-ray result]* were present *[absent]*, how would it change your treatment approach?"

   "Critique the treatment plan proposed by *[another health care provider on the team]*."

   "Compare treatment approach A with treatment approach B."

"Do you think this patient should be _[have been]_ admitted to the hospital? Why or why not?"

"Suggest several potential complications of the most likely diagnosis that we might possibly expect."

"List the critical factors to monitor in the next _[hours, days]_."

Incorporate a Biopsychosocial Approach in Teaching Humanistic Aspects of Patient Care and Medical Education

Teaching the humanistic aspects of patient care seems to be an educational objective that many clinical teachers agree is important, but continues to be neglected in most daily teaching rounds and morning reports. "The need to improve the physician-patient relationship has been recognized for over 50 years. Despite the advent of liaison psychiatry, general hospital psychiatry, and increased teaching of behavioral science in medical school, the integration of psychological and social understanding and skill in medical practice remains fragmentary" (Gorlin & Zucker 1983, p. 1059). Strain and Hamerman (1978) state that "much has been written about humanism and compassion in the approach to the patient, but more specific efforts are needed to educate physicians to manage both mind and body—to practice . . . patient-centered care—which would enhance the physician's skills and more adequately meet the needs of his patients." Teaching humanistic care of patients and teaching about patient care in a humanistic way are really psychomotor skills. As is true for teaching any skill, however, "telling" is not nearly as effective as "doing." The phrase "Don't tell 'em, show 'em" is the critical step in implementing this technique. Mattern and associates (1983) relate the comments of a resident who was impressed with his attending physician's "very deep concern for people's total well-being: physical, emotional, psychological, and spiritual. It is something that you have, and can develop, but it can't be taught except by example."

Engel (1973) has described what he calls "enduring attributes of medicine relevant for the education of the physician." These attributes have remarkably little to do with the possession of biomedical facts or space-age technological skills. In fact, the attribute one might describe as being close to a hard scientific skill is that of "clinical reasoning, judgement, and decision making" (Engel 1973, p. 590), including the thoroughness that McDermott (1982) has described as "the most important element of medical education." Essentially all other attributes are those related to the psychosocial aspects of patient care, attributes like the "complementarity of a need for help and desire to provide service" (p. 588), the critical nature of the interpersonal encounter between the patient and the physician, and the nature of the contract between physician and patient as an interpersonal bond.

Several attempts at more effective teaching of humanistic medicine have been reported (Strain & Hamerman 1978; Frankel & Rosenblum 1983; Gorlin & Zucker 1983). In essentially all cases, these methods have consisted of assigning a psychiatrist or other behavioral medicine specialist to the traditional teaching rounds format. This has been considerably more effective than earlier attempts to merely arrange for the availability of psychiatric liaison services, which fostered a mind-body dichotomy among the house staff. Frankel and Rosenblum (1983) describe a more integrated approach in which psychiatrists regularly attended teaching rounds and participated fully in the patient-based teaching. The success of this approach was almost wholly dependent on the teaching style of the attending "medical" physician. Those attendings who used a biomedically oriented, mini-lecture to discuss mostly the technological aspects of the case did not facilitate the teaching of a biopsychosocial approach to patient care. Their value system was obvious and modeled by the house staff and students.

Another group of attendings recognized the importance of teaching humanistic medical care but were unable to do so themselves. They would defer to the psychiatrist in a helpful but clearly dichotomous way, as if there existed some artificial separation: "Alright, now it's time to talk about the psychiatric aspects of the case." These attendings did change over time, however, so that they scheduled more bedside teaching and more direct interaction with the patient that would allow role modeling of humanistic patient care. "The medical attending, rather than the psychiatrist, . . . would often ask for more psychosocial and mental status exam data in the presentations, and bring up in the discussion "psychiatric" issues such as the relationship between life stresses and the onset or exacerbation of physical symptoms" (Frankel & Rosenblum 1983, p. 137).

The third group of attendings was perhaps the ideal with regard to teaching the psychosocial aspects of patient care. These attendings practiced and taught a totally integrated style of patient care in which psychosocial and biomedical data were considered together and their uses made explicit by the attending. "They took the initiative in asking the house staff to include psychological and social as well as biological data in their presentations, and in highlighting the role of stress in the development of physical illness" (Frankel & Rosenblum 1983, p. 137). For these attendings, the presence of the psychiatrist was perhaps superfluous, and that is, in fact, the goal of teaching the psychosocial aspects of patient care: To incorporate the skills of behavioral specialists so completely that the biomedical and psychosocial aspects of patient care are taught as one, by one attending physician. The ultimate value of behavioral faculty is in the faculty development of medical teachers responsible for medical teaching. This perhaps has been most successful in the specialty of family practice, although considerable conflict regarding the proper role(s) of behavioral faculty still exist (Shapiro, 1980 STFM Task Force, 1985).

Gorlin and Zucker (1983) describe a teaching program based on teaching rounds and morning report that focuses on the emotional reactions of physicians to patients as the basis for learning objectives and teaching activities. The patient situations included terminal illness, incurable disease, emotional crises, and a variety of psychiatric or personality diagnoses such as hostile patients, borderline personalities and dependent and hypochondriacal patients. The physician reactions, which are familiar to any attending physician responsible for teaching rounds, include anger, frustration, guilt, sadness, impatience, disapproval, and feelings of helplessness. The teaching program is built around these difficult physician-patient relationships. Every situation that occurs, in whatever setting (e.g., inpatient service, outpatient clinic, emergency room), is discussed by both a medical and behavioral attending with a series of standard questions of the student or resident:

1. What are you feeling right now about this patient?
2. What is there about this patient, what is he/she doing or saying that causes you to feel this way?
3. What is there about your past experiences or attitudes that contribute to you feeling this way?
4. Can you accept these feelings as valid and real so that we can learn how to cope with them?
5. In what ways can you be helpful and comforting to the patient?
6. Do you have to like the patient before you can be more helpful to him/her?
7. What can you say to this patient whose medical situation makes you feel sad and helpless?
8. What further help for you and the patient might be available from other professionals?
9. Are you able to continue caring for this patient?

The core competencies in psychosocial skills for internal medicine residents have been summarized by Lipkin and associates (1984). These are based on knowledge, attitudes, and skills in the areas of patient-centered interviews and treatment, a biopsychosocial approach to clinical reasoning, the personal development of humanistic attitudes, and specific diagnoses and conditions in psychiatric medicine. This summary, which is highly recommended as a review of this entire field of teaching biopsychosocial and humanistic medicine, describes a number of teaching strategies that are applicable to teaching rounds by the attending physician. These include direct supervision of both brief and extended interviews and patient encounters, role playing, and use of simulated patients (an excellent format for a weekly teaching conference), observation and debriefing of videotapes made of patient interviews by the attending physician, and case conferences and patient presentations discussed in consultation with behavioral faculty.

Perhaps the most effective way of teaching sensitivity to the needs of patients is for the teacher to be sensitive to the needs of the students—a variation of the Golden Rule: "Treat your students as you would have them treat their patients." Attending physicians can be empathetic to the anxieties and fears of medical learners, be patient with their halting efforts to learn, be compassionate about their failures, and be gentle in recognizing their inadequacies, just as attending physicians would be empathetic, patient, compassionate, and gentle with their patients. If learners then can see the attending treating patients in this manner, the instruction will then be complete.

Delegate Teaching and Clinical Responsibilities

This final technique requires the least discussion but is perhaps the most important. The ultimate purpose of any clinical teaching, including that of teaching rounds and morning report, is to bring the learners to a point where they are able to function independently. In fact, the paradox, as stated by Alcott (Auden & Kronenberger 1981), is to "influence learners to be independent of the teacher's influence." Mattern and associates (1983, p. 1131) state that the "importance of transferring the responsibility for teaching to others in the group is consistent with the goal of self-directed learning." In addition to teaching others how to learn and function independently, the attending physician has a responsibility to transfer the teaching function to others, if only for Joubert's (Raimi 1981) well-known but true aphorism, "to teach is to learn twice." To be ultimately successful as an attending physician means moving from a role of solving patient problems and teaching problem solving to a role of watching others do both; i.e., putting oneself out of a job.

Accomplishing this planned obselescence or educational unemployment requires fortitude on the part of the attending. This fortitude is manifested by five characteristics described by Rubeck and Pratt (1979, p. 2):

Tolerance for the ambiguity created by multiple and individual perceptions of purposes, activities, and products;
Committment to growth through individual awareness, to self-knowledge, and to interpersonal experimentation;
A degree of restraint that prevents leaders from imposing their own reactions, thoughts, values, and behavior on other participants;
Empathy for the specific responses made by individual students;
A willingness to wait, while others attend to, interpret, and respond to the discussion in their own perceptions, thoughts, and manner of communication.

The attending physician must make clear at the outset of a teaching rotations that he is there to help the students and residents become independent of his influence, to facilitate the students solving their problems, to provide feedback but not answers, and to provide a forum for critical thinking but not play "Guess What I'm Thinking." The techniques described in chapter 6 (Group Discussions) are applicable to stimulating group critical thinking in a facilitative, rather than coercive, way. Rubeck and Pratt (1979, p. 3, 4) describe several ways that the teacher will know if he has been effective in this regard:

Students will point out inconsistencies or inadequacies in the material presented.

Students will volunteer appropriate information, journal references, or personal experiences when relevant.
Students will ask perceptive questions.
Students will express personal opinions and hypotheses freely.

Tips

A number of specific tips and advice are offered to help implement the techniques described above.

1. Despite its time-consuming nature, a personal meeting with each team member is invaluable for negotiating individual learner needs and clarifying specific patient care responsibilities for each level of student and resident. A follow-up meeting at the end of the rotation is then a natural way to provide (and receive) personal feedback.

2. The attending physician can demand punctuality and committment by demonstrating them himself. The single best predictor of success in teaching rounds is the enthusiasm which the teacher brings to them. The attending can ask at the outset of each meeting the number of new patients and complex "old" patients to be discussed, and divide the available time accordingly, prorating the discussion as it progresses. Learners are much more attentive if they can plan on a specific endpoint to rounds. Arranging for one resident to take all telephone calls will minimize interruptions.

3. Teaching rounds are most effective if case presentations and discussions are their only purpose. Bedside teaching, topic presentations, chart rounds, visits with family members, and team meetings with other health personnel are all valuable, but all of these activities are incompatible in one session. The attending physician may have to schedule separate sessions to accomplish a number of these purposes.

4. Case discussions are most effective if directed mostly at the level of the intern. This level of learning will be stimulating to the students,

and higher-level residents can be brought in as teachers by asking them to critique opinions and fill gaps in information. Students can be assigned library research at the end of each discussion for presentation at the next meeting. Blackboards are particularly helpful for "on the spot" audiovisual help.

5. Individual chart rounds by the attending physician are a valuable supplement of information about student and resident performance. This also provides an opportunity for the attending to give honest positive feedback early in the rotation, so that negative feedback can be given, when necessary, with greater comfort.

6. The attending should often play the role of "devil's advocate" so as to stimulate learner participation and critical thinking. A useful goal for pacing discussions and participation is for the attending to talk less than one-third of the time.

7. A final trick that helps establish the clinical credibility so critical to the success of the attending physician is to arrange to be clinically visible by scheduling call assignments and clinic schedules appropriately. In the absence of these opportunities, the liberal use of "war stories" is almost as valuable.

Conclusion

Efficient and effective management of formal teaching conferences and morning report is a sophisticated skill requiring considerable enthusiasm, interpersonal ability, negotiating skill, and dedication, in addition to the requisite medical knowledge. In its most highly refined form, an excellent teaching rounds session is one of the most potent forms of clinical teaching possible. That such powerful experiences are infrequently found in today's medical education is more a result of a lack of faculty time, energy, and reward for teaching, than because of a lack of teaching ability. Physician teachers who take on major responsibility for this type of teaching may find that the skills and behaviors described in this chapter are already a part of their repertoire, if only subconsciously. To bring them to a level of usefulness requires only a willingness to do so, along with good intentions towards their students, and a bit of common sense. A commitment to learner needs, similar to a physician's commitment to patient needs, and the commitment to learners as individuals with specific past experiences and future objectives will serve physician teachers well.

CHAPTER 8

Bedside Teaching

There should be "no teaching without a patient for a text, and the best teaching is that taught by the patient himself." (Osler 1903)

Perhaps in no other area of medical teaching are the stated desires of physician faculty more discrepant with reality than in bedside teaching. If we were to ask almost any physician faculty member how important it is to teach at the bedside, the answer would likely be positive and effusive: "There is nothing more important in the education of young physicians than to go to the bedside of patients with the attending physician." Yet if we then asked residents and students how frequently did experienced attending physicians take them to the bedside, the answer would be, "Nearly never!". Payson and Barchas (1965), in a study of ward medical teaching, found that less than 20% of teaching time was spent in the presence of the patient, and most of that was spent by the attending physician performing his own physical examination. Collins and associates (1978) reported similar findings 13 years later. No evidence suggests that the situation has reversed itself more recently; yet surveys of students and residents regarding the characteristics of teaching and teachers they find most valuable list items such as "empathetic," "compassionate," "gentle," "demonstrates concern for the patient," and "interested in psychosocial needs of patients" (Stritter et al. 1975; Irby 1978; Lamkin et al. 1983). These characteristics can only be demonstrated at the bedside. Studies of the competencies of students and residents in taking accurate histories and performing appropriate physical examinations suggest that significant errors occur in over 50% of complete evaluations observed (Wiener & Nathanson 1976). Most students and residents report completing their medical training rarely having been observed performing full bedside evaluations of patients.

The purpose of this chapter is to help the physician in extending his repertoire of clinical teaching skills to teaching at the bedside in a way that is comfortable and productive. Previous studies describe several barriers that discourage clinical teachers from teaching at the bedside:

Concern for the privacy and dignity of the patient;
A lack of skills in interacting simultaneously with the student and the patient;
The view that medical education is a passive process that best occurs in the classroom, where students are not involved in medical decision making;
The discomfort that clinical teachers have in dealing with a broad array of subjects and concerns usually raised at the bedside.

This chapter will extend the physician's natural skills of patient interaction to the new domain of teacher-learner-patient interactions. In the process, these four barriers will be found to be readily overcome or to be educationally spurious.

Objectives

There are four fundamental objectives of any bedside teaching interaction:

1. To base all teaching on data generated by or about the patient;
2. To conduct bedside rounds with respect for the patient's comfort and dignity;
3. To use bedside teaching particularly for teaching psychomotor skills;
4. To use every opportunity in bedside teaching to provide feedback to learners.

The first objective might seem at first thought to be obvious and trivial. It is obvious; it is far from trivial. The only purpose of bedside teaching is to teach knowledge, attitudes, and skills related directly to the patient at hand. The simplicity of this purpose may be missed by some bedside teachers who are unwittingly drawn into tangential discussions, making the patient's presence only vaguely helpful. Also, some teachers may consider the patient to be someone whose purpose is to be impressed by the depth and breadth of the teacher's eloquent soliloquy on matters that may not always pertain to the patient's case. In both cases, the patient is confused, the learners embarrassed, and the value of the patient's presence is lost. Although over 300 years old, the advice of Sylvius, the 17th century chair of medicine at Leiden, is still valid regarding the focus of bedside teaching:

> My method . . . [is to] lead my students by the hand to the practice of medicine, taking them every day to see patients in the public hospital, that they may hear the patient's symptoms and see their physical findings. (Linfors & Neelon 1980, p. 1231)

In most cases, teaching should focus on history, physical examination findings, or psychomotor skills being taught, or should be used as an opportunity to demonstrate appropriate methods of patient interaction and consideration for the psychosocial aspects of patient care. Hurst (1971, p. 464) notes the "the time physicians and students spend with patients should be devoted entirely to the patient. Each patient is unique and what each says and reveals must be listened to and studied carefully."

The second objective, that of conducting bedside teaching with respect for the patient's comfort and dignity, benefits both patient and learners. For the patient, bedside rounds can be an opportunity for the attending physician to publicly (as opposed to privately, with only the patient present) demonstrate his concern for the patient's emotional state, and to empathize with the anxiety and distress felt by the patient regarding his medical situation. This public display can often enhance even the most positive physician-patient relationship and provides the physician the opportunity to rectify relationships that may be somewhat tenuous because of a particularly traumatic disease or treatment. Romano (1941, p. 667) notes that "ward round teaching, when conducted tactfully and sympathetically . . . is not a traumatic emotional experience to patients, but educates and reassures them." Linfors and Neelon (1980) found that 95% of patients felt bedside rounds were a positive experience.

For residents and students, demonstrating respect for the patient's emotional comfort is as educationally powerful as demonstrating a complex psychomotor skill. In fact, the psychosocial aspects of patient care are so complex that the *only* way and place that they may be taught is by demonstrating psychosocial techniques of interaction while learners observe directly at the bedside. To tell a student or resident how to demonstrate concern and caring is fruitless, or (even worse) may trivialize one of the most critical criteria of professional success. In a study of effective attending physician teaching behaviors a resident comments on the critical contribution made by one attending physician (Mattern et al. 1983, p. 1131): "He has this very deep concern for people's total well-being: physical, emotional, psychological, and spiritual. It is something that you have, and can develop, but it can't be taught except by example."

Demonstrating concern for the patient's psychosocial status, then, has a double payoff in both better patient care and critical teaching that can be done in no other way.

The importance of basing all bedside teaching on patient-related data and issues has already been stressed. This importance includes using bedside teaching as a critical time for the teaching of psychomotor skills. These skills include the usual diagnostic and therapeutic procedures, such as venipuncture, catheter insertion, and lumbar puncture, but also include physical examination skills and medical problem solving skills. The former seems more obviously a psychomotor procedure, but the latter is a skill that requires demonstration and practice just as does a surgical procedure. In fact, the mistake often made in teaching clinical problem solving is that it is described and "practiced" in a vacuum—in the absence of the patient whose problem is being solved. The techniques of teaching psychomotor and surgical skills apply as well, and perhaps even better, to the skill of problem solving. The study by Weiner and Nathanson (1976) shows that students and residents are observed and critiqued performing physical examinations with remarkable infrequency. While the outcome of problem solving is paid considerable attention, the process probably receives as little attention as does the performance of the physical examination—the bedside is the perfect, and only, place to rectify both of these educational deficiencies.

An important learning objective of bedside rounds, which cannot be achieved as well by many other teaching formats, is evaluation by the teacher of the learner. Giving both positive and negative feedback is a critical part of the bedside teacher's job. Feedback has formative and summative purposes (described in chapter 4), and both have value at the bedside. Feedback is only valuable if the knowledge about the learner is detailed and intimate—the bedside is the best place to obtain it. Ultimately the only feedback worth giving is that which concerns the care of patients. Attempts to do otherwise will be inaccurate at best, hollow and trivial at worst. When the physician-teacher wishes to truly understand the patient care abilities of his students or residents, bedside teaching is the only place to be.

Techniques

The techniques helpful to the clinician who wants to be a better bedside teacher can be organized according the four objectives of bedside teaching:

1. Basing all teaching on patient data;
2. Conducting bedside teaching with respect for the comfort of the patient;
3. Capitalizing on bedside teaching as an opportunity to teach psychomotor skills;
4. Using bedside teaching as a special opportunity to give learners feedback.

Techniques for giving feedback effectively have been presented in chapter 4; techniques for accomplishing the first three objectives are presented here.

Base all Bedside Teaching on Patient Data

To extend the previous quotation from Sylvius, "I question the students as to what they have noted in the patients and about their thoughts and perceptions regarding the cause of the illnesses and the principles of treatment" (Linfors & Neelon 1980, p. 1231). The point of going to the patient's bedside is to have access to and direct observation of patient data: The history in the patient's own words, physical examination data collected by the teacher and learners, a negotiated style of clinical problem solving in which steps in the process are checked with the patient and conclusions agreed upon, and opportunities for demonstrating and practicing bedside psychomotor procedures. Hurst (1971, p. 464) notes the bulk of the patient presentation should not be made in the presence of the patient but should adequately prepare the learners to benefit maximally from the time spent with the patient: "The time physicians and students spend with patients should be devoted entirely to the patient. Each patient is unique and what each says and reveals must be listened to and studied carefully." This means that case presentations, either complete or partial, must be made succinctly, that all data bearing on a particular problem be presented together, that not all problems necessarily be discussed, that the presenter give a clear overview of the patient's situation, that the purpose of subsequently visiting the patient be specified, and that time be allowed for questions between presentation and patient visit so that no confusion or ambiguity persists. Should the discussion or activity waver from a patient-based focus, the attending physician has the choice of concluding that "the point of diminishing returns" has been reached and can bring the bedside teaching to a close, or can reassert (publicly) the need to return to the issue at hand: the patient and his immediate care and concerns. This has indirect benefits in demonstrating again and with certainty for the patient his central importance to the teacher's thinking and that of the residents and students.

Conduct Bedside Teaching With Concern for Patient's Comfort and Dignity

Osler's method of bedside teaching is as applicable today as in the early 1900s, as indicated by a description by one of his students:

> [Osler] would go to the patient's bed, stand (or sometimes sit in a chair) near the head of the bed at the patient's right side,

give him a cheery greeting and, if he were a new patient, ask for his history . . . After it had been commented on . . . and often added to and illuminated by Dr. Osler with accompanying pertinent remarks, the report of the physical examination was called for from the clinical clerk . . . Usually Dr. Osler made some examination himself and demonstrated and discussed patient features, all the time mingling his discussion with remarks and explanations to the patient, so that he would not be mystified or frightened . . . Often, patients whose cases had previously been discussed were passed over quickly, but Dr. Osler never failed to give some bright, cheering words to the patient. (Christian, 1949, pp. 81-82)

Linfors and Neelon (1980, p. 1231) found that 95% of patients saw bedside rounds as a positive experience, but that patients had several suggestions for improvement: "They wanted the attending physician to introduce himself, to state the purpose of bedside rounds, and to be sensitive to the need to translate technical terms. They also thought that the patient should receive advance notice of bedside rounds and that rounds should not be so long as to tire the patient." Hurst notes that the presenter, who should know the patient best, should visit the patient after rounds to clarify misunderstandings and relieve any anxieties created by rounds. Also, Hurst (1971, p. 464) reinforces Osler's technique of leaving the bedside "with an optimistic statement of some sort even if it is no more than stating that the physicians caring for the patient are working diligently on the patient's problems." This last statement has the additional value of reinforcing the legitimacy of the patient care provided by the residents and students and enhances their professional position in the eyes of the patient.

In summary, bedside teaching can be productive for learners and respectful of patients if these guidelines are followed:

1. Common human courtesy guides the asking of patient permission and the introduction of teacher, learners and the proposed activities;
2. Physical examinations and procedures are performed and practiced with appropriate explanation, as a physician would do in normal patient care circumstances;
3. All conversations, information transfer, and technical discussions are made in a way that the patient is included and understands;
4. The patient is actively engaged in a three-way dialogue with the teacher and learners regarding the medical problem solving process, with conclusions (tentative or firm, and so stated) made clearly to the patient;
5. A resident or student sees the patient afterward, perhaps during usual work rounds, to clarify questions, concerns, and misconceptions, and bring the teaching event to a productive close.

Use Bedside Teaching Opportunities to Demonstrate and Practice Medical and Surgical Procedures

Some medical teachers erroneously imagine that clinical skills and procedures can be taught in the absence of a patient or without the opportunity to practice these procedures in a clinical setting. Demonstrations, lectures, videotape presentations, or reading cannot substitute for the opportunity of an experienced clinician demonstrating procedures to students with a patient, and then allowing the students to practice in a way that does not compromise quality patient care. Bedside teaching is just such an opportunity, and perhaps the best. Residents may take junior house staff and students to the bedside during their work rounds, and the patient may be seen during teaching rounds and attending physician morning report, but a concentrated time devoted to learning patient procedures at the bedside has no substitute.

Psychomotor skills traditionally have been learned according to the old surgical dictum, "See one, do one, teach one." With one modification, educational research actually supports this as a valid, if terse, aphorism for the teaching of skills. The modification includes a bit more emphasis on practice, so that a more valid and educationally sound dictum would be, "See one, do one, *do one more,* teach one." Specific techniques to implement this advice include teaching skills at the level of the learner and using the methods of "backward chaining" or "forward lengthening" (see Introductory Phase) to teach sequential skills.

Learners progress through four levels of sophistication as they learn new skills (Personnel Journal, 1974). Teachers must be aware of the level of sophistication at which a learner is currently functioning and match their teaching to that level. Teaching at a level of understanding that is higher or lower than that of the learner is unproductive and/or frustrating. The four levels of understanding through which learners pass in becoming competent practitioners of a skill are

1. Unconsciously incompetent;
2. Consciously incompetent;
3. Consciously competent;
4. Unconsciously competent.

Most learners start at level 1, where they do not even know what they do not know. Most teachers are at level 4, where they can "do it in their sleep." The teacher must join the learner, since the converse situation is impossible. For example, in teaching a junior medical student, who is *unconsciously incompetent,* how to draw a venous blood specimen, the teacher would first make the learner aware of the technique's existence, the equipment required, and the indications and contraindications. The learner would then know what he does not know and be *consciously incompetent.* Proper demonstration and practice on models, fellow learners and patients would allow the learner to see and perform the procedure incorrectly, albeit with hesitation and anxiety, and thus become _consciously competent._ Hundreds of correct performances later, the learner would be _unconsciously competent._ In moving from level 1 to level 4, the learner moves through three phases. The teacher can use the following 12 steps (which includes an example of teaching the skill of venipuncture) to help the learner progress from level 1 to level 4.

Introductory Phase ("See One"). 1. State the objective of the skill teaching about to be done and the specific performance that is expected at the conclusion of the teaching: "The objective of this session is to teach you how to perform a venipuncture for the purpose of obtaining laboratory blood specimens, and I expect you to perform one venipuncture satisfactorily at the conclusion of the session."

2. Explain the rationale and importance of the skill: "Venipuncture is a common procedure done in hospitals and offices, and you will be asked frequently as medical students to obtain blood for various laboratory tests."

3. Present a description of the necessary equipment and materials, and an overview of the skill's basic sequential steps: "The equipment necessary to perform a venipuncture are shown here. . . . The first step is to select a site of venous access, usually the antecubital fossa. . . ."

4. Explain how each sequential step is done: "The next step is to apply a tourniquet on the upper arm, using this rubber strap or a blood pressure cuff inflated to a pressure between the diastolic and systolic pressure."

5. Demonstrate the entire skill, using the technique of either _backward chaining_ or _forward lengthening._ Many medical and surgical procedures are actually a series of sequential steps, each of which must be performed correctly and in proper sequence. In order to teach these procedures effectively, it is important that they be broken into their discrete components rather than taught as an indigestible lump. In backward chaining, the last step is demonstrated and practiced first to give learners a sense of the procedure's endpoint and outcome.

Each preceding step is then demonstrated and practiced, followed in sequence by the latter steps already learned. This procedure works well for lengthy procedures, the endpoints and outcomes of which are not immediately obvious to learners. Forward lengthening is the opposite of backward chaining. The first step is demonstrated and practiced first, and subsequent steps are added until the last step is reached. This method works well for short procedures, such as venipuncture, that have readily apparent outcomes: "The last step, which I'm performing now, is to apply an absorbent gauze or cotton ball to the site and flex the elbow so as to achieve hemostasis."

The learner has now progressed to level 2, consciously incompetent, and can proceed to the practice phase.

Practice Phase ("Do One").   6. Give specific instructions on what to practice and how: "I'd like you to begin by choosing a partner, laying out your equipment, and demonstrating to me the vein you will be using for this venipuncture."

7. Observe and practice closely and give frequent brief promptings about how the learner is doing: "The arm should be more extended, and the tourniquet a bit tighter."

8. Provide generous quantities of feedback generated by the learner, his peers, and the instructor (in that order): "Tell me how you think you did in explaining to the patient what you were about to do."

9. Allow a period of independent practice time: "I'll be out of the room for about 15 minutes and want each of you to perform a complete venipuncture by the time I get back."

10. Certify each student on the entire skill: "Over the next 2 days, each of you should come and get me to watch you do an entire venipuncture."

The student has now progressed to level 3, consciously competent, and can move on to the perfecting phase.

Perfecting Phase ("Do One More").   11. Provide precision practice under realistic stress situations: "During the next 4 weeks of your clerkship, I want you to perform 10 venipunctures needed by your ward team."

12. Prompt and give feedback only rarely: "The last three veni-punctures you did seemed to go quite well. I noticed this time that you seemed a bit unsteady in collecting the second tube of blood."

The student has now progressed to level 4, unconsciously compe-tent, and is able to "teach one."

Tips

A number of brief teaching tips, collected from experienced bed-side teachers, may be useful in supplementing the techniques de-scribed in the preceding section.

1. A frequent problem for teachers is the confusion that results when bedside teaching is incorporated with morning report and more formal attending rounds or team teaching rounds. Separating the two types of teaching, which really have different objectives and a differ-ent style, may improve both types of teaching. Scheduling a distinct time for demonstrating physical findings, interviewing a particularly difficult patient, or teaching a specific procedure may be much more productive.

2. Bedside teaching is often harder to do with learners of markedly different levels of experience, unless the teacher is adept at using learners more experienced to teach those who are not. Scheduling bedside teaching with learners of similar experience, such as medical students, while excluding others, such as interns, may be helpful.

3. Patients who are somewhat reluctant to participate in bedside teaching will become much more enthused if approached by the phy-sician closest to them (whether student or attending) who can empha-size the important educational role to be played by the patient.

4. The comfort level of both patient and learner may be increased by demonstrating certain techniques or procedures (such as physical examination techniques) on a learner first. This is especially true for pediatric patients.

5. The patient with chronic disease or longstanding findings can often be used as the teacher by asking him to describe certain physical findings or abnormalities best known to him. (For an excellent discussion of the great educational value of developing patients as trained instructors, see Stillman et al. 1980.)

6. It is possible to give learners feedback in the presence of the patient (the most valuable but riskiest way to do it) by asking a learner for his opinion about a diagnosis or treatment, acknowledging the correct portions of his answer, and incorporating them in the summation to the patient. When incorporating these answers, the learner receives "credit" for the correct portions while realizing those portions not acknowledged are thought to be less useful or accurate by the teacher: "Mr. Jones, I think student Dr. Smith is absolutely correct about the mitral valve causing your heart murmur. I do think, however, that you have mostly mitral stenosis, rather than mitral insufficiency, causing your problems."

7. The use of humor is absolutely critical for the teacher serving as a ringleader for a patient and a group of learners. Embarassing moments, learner mistakes, lengthy demonstrations, and inappropriate behaviors (by any of the parties involved) are handled well by gentle humor, philosophic comments, and kind words.

8. The teacher is sometimes well served by being able to say "I don't know." Demonstrating the need to pursue further information about a problem, finding, or complication is educationally sound, intellectually honest, and, in the long run, therapeutic for the patient who will trust the attending physician who is willing to acknowledge the need to pursue a problem in greater depth (Herwig, 1986).

Conclusion

In summary, bedside teaching is an enriching, and intimate form of teaching that offers unmatched opportunities to the physician teacher for directly demonstrating procedures, directly observing learner skills, and giving immediate substantive feedback to learners . Medical education has crowded out this type of clinical teaching format from most curriculi, to the detriment of both learners and teachers. There are specific techniques of bedside teaching, as there are for all teaching formats, that can make it efficient, productive, and satisfying. Ultimately, the teacher behavior that most predicts the success of the bedside teacher is acknowledging and maintaining the proper balance between patient and learner needs.

CHAPTER 9

Clinical Teaching in the Ambulatory Setting

The teaching of clinical medicine in ambulatory settings may well be an idea
whose time has finally come. (Perkoff, 1986)
Learning primary care medicine in a university hospital is like trying to learn
forestry in a lumberyard. (Anon., in Verby et al. 1981)

   Most of the teaching skills described in chapters 5–8 apply to teaching that takes place in the classroom or the hospital, for the simple
reason that most medical education traditionally has taken place in
the classroom or the hospital. The post-Flexner era of medical education and the post–World War II era of scientific medical practice are
characterized by medical care that is technologically based, by caring
for patients in the hospital where the technology is available, and by
teaching where the patients are (i.e., the hospital), or where the basic
sciences of medical technology can be most easily taught (i.e., the
classroom). Recently, however, several new forces are causing the
locus of medical care in the academic medical center, and therefore
the locus of some portions of medical education, to shift to the ambulatory and primary care sector (Schwenk & Detmer 1986). (The terms
"ambulatory care" and "primary care" are not necessarily synonomous, but for the purposes of this discussion, they will be considered

so. However, even the teaching of cardiothoracic surgery in the surgery clinic may benefit from the use of some of the skills described in this chapter.) Perkoff (1986) has summarized the reasons that ambulatory care teaching is becoming a more important component of the total medical education process: Less inpatients available for teaching purposes due to a decreased number of hospital admissions and shorter lengths of stay, the ability to provide in an ambulatory setting much of the care previously provided in the hospital, the demand by health maintenance organizations (HMOs) and other large, structured medical care delivery systems for physicians expert in the delivery of high-quality and efficient ambulatory care, and the need for hospitals to establish and staff ambulatory care centers to "capture" patients requiring inpatient care. For these reasons, and others, specific skills in ambulatory care teaching are necessary to guarantee the quality of the educational process. However, since ambulatory medical care differs greatly from inpatient care, teaching in the two locations is very different. The types of activities, the learning objectives, and the resultant teaching skills are unique to the type of care provided and the setting in which it is provided. This chapter will begin by describing types of ambulatory teaching activities, before (as was done in previous chapters) describing learning objectives and the teaching techniques to meet those objectives.

Types of Ambulatory Teaching Activities

Unlike inpatient medical education, which has certain commonalities and traditions no matter the specialty and specific unit, ambulatory teaching takes on as many forms as there are types of outpatient care. For both students and residents, ambulatory experiences can occur in private medical offices; large group medical organizations and HMOs; model resident training centers in family medicine; physician-directed outpatient clinics in general internal medicine, pediatrics, and obstetrics-gynecology; outpatient subspecialty clinics; emergency departments and urgent care centers; and community agencies such as family planning and health department well-child clinics.

Primary care experiences for medical students have been organized as intense rotational clerkships; part-time longitudinal assignments in private offices; primary care tracks that include several ambulatory activities during the course of medical school; and integrated, long-term, full-time primary care preceptorial experiences. Representative examples of these are described next. Blumenthal and colleagues (1983) described a particular community preceptorship program in primary care that included these specific objectives:

To provide experiences in critically examining the physician-patient relationship and interaction;

To facilitate understanding of providing primary care to underserved patient populations;

To allow students to construct patient and family profiles through interviews;

To familiarize students with the breadth of primary care problems;

To expose students to the nonmedical aspects of medical practice;

To provide experience in taking histories and performing physical examinations in the ambulatory setting.

To accomplish these objectives, students spent a half-day per month with a preceptor during the first 2 years of medical school. Preceptor sites were rotated monthly to widen exposure.

Grover and associates (1977) described a didactic and clinical curriculum for first-year students that focused on HMO-based care. Seminars and brief preceptorships were used throughout the one-term course to accomplish objectives related to learning about the system of providing capitated care. Students also followed the care of one patient, including making home visits. The University of Iowa provided an extensive set of required and elective full-time, community-based preceptorships for third- and fourth-year medical students (Caplan 1975). The program was part of a primary care track designed to "capture" an increased number of students practicing primary care in rural Iowa communities after residency training.

Becker and Stillman (1981) described a 2-week, full-time community-based pediatric clerkship that utilized day care centers, schools, residential centers, detention facilities, and private practices to give students the "opportunity to interview and examine a diverse population of children of all ages from a wide variety of nationalities, socioeconomic backgrounds, and cultural heritages." Students were exposed to pediatric patients with both acute and chronic illnesses, but the experience emphasized behavioral and health maintenance issues.

Beasley (1983) has described an "academically intensive third-year three-month family practice clerkship based in private practice settings." Compared with other experiences, this experience is designed to meet the clinical objectives of clinical medical students (as opposed to more introductory experiences for preclinical students) by basing the clerkships in carefully selected private practices. Preceptors (called "tutors" in this program) were also carefully selected, and pursued specific faculty development activities. The preceptorships had specific objectives that were analogous to those of traditional third-year clerkships based in teaching hospitals, although the objectives were not identical since ambulatory patients were used to meet those objectives.

Olness (1975) described another alternative clerkship for ambulatory teaching that used the pediatric facilities of a university-based HMO. The goals for the clerkship were to

1. Provide an example of high-quality ambulatory care;
2. Teach techniques for collecting and recording ambulatory data;
3. Foster appropriate attitudes in students towards the physician-patient relationship;
4. Teach students about systems of health care delivery.

Four or five students were incorporated into health care teams that included two staff pediatricians, a nurse practitioner, and a receptionist. Each student saw several patients during a half-day, and learned routine office laboratory skills and techniques. Students also had brief lectures and other small-group didactic experiences during the clerkship. The staff pediatricians responsible for the students were partially supported by the medical school (20% of salary) to compensate for presumed decreased efficiency.

Pawlson and associates (1979) described a similar clerkship for third-year students in general internal medicine. These students spent eight weeks in ambulatory settings, rotating through a university-sponsored HMO, private offices, and ambulatory-based subspecialty clinics and emergency departments. Whenever appropriate, the students functioned as members of the primary care team. A careful cost-accounting mechanism showed that the total cost per student per day of this varied ambulatory care experience was $54.20, for a total of approximately $11,500/student/year. The bulk of this cost (64%) was for faculty time, but nonfaculty personnel costs, space, and materials also contributed a third of the total. Pawlson and associates (1979, p. 555) calculate that the yearly costs for a full-time, 8-week clerkship for a class of 150 third-year students would be approximately $300,000, and that "the structure of clinical instruction in U.S. medical schools generates such high costs since it relies on small groups and/or one-to-one teaching using relatively expensive instructors (physicians)."

More intense, time-consuming experiences also exist for medical students. Putnam and colleagues (1975) described a 2-month experience in which a senior medical student replaced a family nurse practitioner in a rural health center. The health center was staffed by family nurse practitioners, community health workers, and part-time physicians in internal medicine, pediatrics, obstetrics, and psychiatry. Physicians provided direct patient care as well as direct and indirect supervision of ancillary medical personnel.

"The student quickly settled into the routine of a nurse practitioner. Early in the morning he met with the two community health workers to discuss patients seen in the health center the previous day; the community health workers informed the student of the problems they had encountered during their home visits. Together the student and community health workers developed plans for the day. Following this, the student saw patients at the health center, made home visits with a community health worker, or met with one of the physicians to review patients" (Putnam et al. 1975, p. 285). The student felt that he acquired an understanding of the following aspects of primary care practice:

1. The natural history of common medical problems;
2. The relationship of psychosocial and family data to biomedical illness;
3. The value and availability of health care resources outside the health center;
4. The diagnosis and treatment of common medical problems, and the importance of the health care team in primary care delivery.

Another important experiment in the intense teaching of ambulatory and primary care is the Rural Physician Associate Program (RPAP) of the University of Minnesota Medical School (Verby et al. 1981). The RPAP was designed to partially solve the following problems with ambulatory medical education:

Intense competition for clinical experiences in hospitals and clinics with too many students and too few patients;

The lack of opportunity to see the value of continuity of medical care and to observe the progress of a patient through an illness;

The infrequency with which a student experiences an intense, long-term relationship with a medical teacher who can accurately assess and help remedy a student's weaknesses and deficiencies;

The inability of students to have a realistic view of primary care from usual medical school rotations.

The RPAP provides a 9- to 12-month, full-time experience for third-year medical students in a community-based private practice. "Students and their families live in the community and work with selected primary care physicians and their colleagues, gaining full exposure to the role of a primary care physician. Their curriculum is supplemented throughout the entire preceptorship by visits from a variety of university specialists" (Verby et al., 1981, p. 646). Students in RPAP experiences logged an average of 344 patient encounters per month, compared with 115 patient encounters per month for a control group of medical students assigned to the usual medical center clerkships. Standardized cognitive testing, such as national board examinations, showed equal performance by the two groups.

In summary, an incredible variety of primary care and ambulatory care experiences have been developed, with essentially similar objectives. Evaluations of programs, participating students and financial costs show high-volume experiences of high academic and clinical quality, with attendent financial costs that are often prohibitive without outside financial support. These undergraduate experiences naturally lead to needs for strong ambulatory teaching at the residency level. Charney (1975, p. 129) notes that "in the last few years an intense amount of discussion, hand-wringing, and even some program changes have taken place in residency education for primary practice." He also notes that essentially all efforts to strengthen ambulatory teaching of residents take on two forms: either a continuity model practice beginning in the first year of training such as that used in family practice, or a traditional internship followed by more intense ambulatory rotational experiences of varying lengths and with varying amounts of interspersed inpatient training. In either type of residency ambulatory training, the goals appear to be the same; the training provides these opportunities:

1. Experience with patients from a more representative cross-section of the community than may be seen in a hospital outpatient department;
2. Further development of the doctor's interview skills;
3. Experience with longitudinal management of chronic disease and with preventive services;
4. Experience with unselected acute or common illnesses;
5. Study of a functional primary care organization (i.e., administration, patient flow, medical records, costs, and, less commonly, the effect of consumer input);
6. Involvement with nurse practitioners or other middle-level health personnel;
7. Continuous responsibility for first-contact medicine (24-hour on-call system);
8. Experience with the milieu of practice (to be contrasted with the milieu of the hospital).

A number of different ambulatory experiences have been tested to meet all or part of these objectives. Greenberg (1979) described a rotation in which pediatric residents were assigned to a brief outpatient experience in the offices of solo pediatricians or those of a group pediatric practice. Practices were carefully selected for medical quality and educational enthusiasm. The experience lasted only 2 weeks but received high evaluations from all parties involved, including private patients and their parents.

Goodson and associates (1980) described a somewhat different rotation in internal medicine, in which residents rotated through a number of ambulatory clinics over a 5-week period, including some continuity experience in a general medical clinic. "Rounds" were held in which all or most ambulatory patients seen during a session were presented and discussed. Financial analyses suggested that 90% of expenses could be covered if residents saw six patients per session in the general medical clinic.

A similar experience was developed in a Veterans' Administration hospital (Casciato et al. 1979); the goals of this continuity care clinic were

1. To provide continuity of medical care of veteran patients discharged from the acute care medical wards;
2. To provide outpatient medical consultations for surgery, dermatology, neurology, and rehabilitation medicine services and to give house staff members experience as office-based general medical consultants;
3. To provide experience for house staff members in the continuing primary care of outpatients;
4. To provide an environment for the teaching of ambulatory care;
5. To provide an environment suitable for research in ambulatory care.

Residents in internal medicine were scheduled for 1 full day/week of Internal Medicine Clinic (IMC), during which senior and junior residents practiced together, a literature file was readily available, faculty physicians provided direct and indirect supervision, and charts were reviewed randomly for quality of care criteria. An evaluation of resident reactions and satisfaction showed that most patients seen had common medical illnesses, that the IMC provided educational opportunities not otherwise available in traditional inpatient rotations, and that 90% of residents thought the rotation was satisfactory or better. Of particular value to the residents was the experience of providing continuity of care, of being able to follow patients discharged from the hospital, and of learning to deal with types of problems not normally seen in traditional subspecialty clinics.

Lipsitz (1982), who completed primary care, internal medicine training that included several community-based ambulatory experiences, reported a much different experience. These activities occurred on a part-time longitudinal basis, with more intense, full-time experiences interspersed. In addition to accomplishing objectives similar to those already described, Lipsitz (1982, p. 25–26) described certain less tangible, but critical, learning achievements:

> In my community experience, patients were on their own turf, responsible for their own care, and capable of accepting or rejecting privately what I had to offer. The patient clearly had control, and only he or she could decide whether to pursue certain investigations, take prescribed medications, or heed a physician's advice. The process of patient education, physician-patient interaction, careful listening, and risk-benefit analysis became more important than facts and figures. I learned to deal with uncertainty and ambiguity in formulating a diagnosis and had to understand the patient's psychosocial and cultural background in order to implement a treatment plan. Sometimes time was the best tool for diagnosis and nonintervention the best treatment. Such an attitude can be taught in any outpatient setting, so long as the focus is shifted from technology and disease to individual patients and their expectations. Community experience can provide a humbling perspective on the doctor-patient relationship.

Both the medical and psychosocial objectives described above have been incorporated into a primary care internal medicine program described by Goroll and colleagues (1975). The ambulatory teaching objectives include the diagnosis and treatment of acute adult medical problems, the evaluation and management of chronic diseases, including the attendant emotional and social issues, the practice of preventive medicine, the understanding of peer review, the organization and operation of a health care team, and the psychosocial aspects of the physician-patient relationship. Several activities accomplish these objectives, including the organization of the residents and faculty physicians into health care teams responsible for a panel of patients, the scheduling of physicians so that a member of the team is always available, and the holding of daily "visit rounds" at which all new patients, and difficult followup patients, are presented for detailed discussions of diagnosis, treatment and management, and behavioral issues. Patients are often videotaped, or directly interviewed at these rounds. Medical and psychosocial consultants are sometimes present. The team also holds ambulatory work rounds at which all ambulatory patients are presented for discussions by residents, faculty supervisors, social workers, and nurses. Supervision of patient care is provided directly by faculty physicians for all patients seen, and charts are audited frequently and randomly. Several different didactic presentations are made, including weekly Ambulatory Grand Rounds and thrice weekly seminars on nonmedical aspects of ambulatory care. Residents are evaluated by faculty through direct observation, case discussions, and chart review. A similar, although less well-developed, educational model in obstetrics and gynecology has been described by Tatelbaum et al. (1978).

Proger (1975) has described a far more ambitious model for generic ambulatory training that markedly deemphasizes hospital training and includes premedical education in the humanities and behavioral sciences, a decreased time commitment to basic biomedical sciences, a lengthened and more narrowly focused clinical training in ambulatory medical care in all its forms (subspecialty clinics, emergency departments, primary care centers, community health centers, and private offices), and an ambulatory care externship that is the equivalent of the usual inpatient internship.

Family practice residency training is heavily based on ambulatory teaching; its format varies but is usually based on a faculty-resident team concept of care that provides longitudinal experiences for residents throughout the entire three years of residency training. Other variations include resident-only teams supervised by faculty who maintain a private practice elsewhere, and a model of training that is almost entirely outpatient in the second and third years of training with interspersed brief rotations in ambulatory subspecialties (the nonrotational "Sparrow" model of training, (Crow et al. 1980). Ambulatory teaching is done in the usual fashion, with direct faculty supervision, videotape debriefing, intensive precepting in which behavioral and medical faculty directly observe residents with patients, chart audits, end-of-session conferences in which some or all patients are presented and discussed, case conferences, role playing, and computer assisted training in clinical problem solving. The main difference between this system and that described above by Goroll and colleagues is that family practice training has as the focus of teaching and unit of care the family rather than the individual patient (Schwenk & Hughes 1983).

Comparison of Ambulatory and Inpatient Teaching

What is common to all of these varied ambulatory experiences? What generalizations can be made to help define the objectives and techniques of ambulatory teaching? Perkoff (1986) describes several differences in ambulatory teaching that distinguish it from inpatient teaching. Inpatient teaching has considerable tradition and precedence—learner responsibilities for patient evaluations and presentations are clear. Inpatient teaching is scheduled, occurs in groups, and problems are discussed in depth. Ambulatory teaching, on the other hand, usually involves one teacher and one learner discussing one patient briefly, in whatever breadth is necessary, on an unscheduled basis that accomodates patient flow demands and unscheduled visits. The patient is available only briefly, reading and preparation before presentation and discussion are impossible, formal rounds are infrequent, and patients exercise considerable control over what they do and when they do it. On the other hand, issues concerning the physician-patient relationship and interaction are more easily taught because of their immediate importance, and psychosocial factors are more prominent and visible factors requiring attention since the patient is closer to his own "turf." Patients are less complex biomedically but more complex psychosocially.

The logistical issues are similar to those in inpatient teaching, except that faculty time is often poorly utilized. If too many learners are seeing and requiring supervision of too many patients, the faculty is overloaded and medical care suffers. The opposite situation means that the faculty's attention often wanders to other more pressing concerns. Learner needs are similar, in that they want participation and responsibility and hope that both will increase with their level of experience. Learners want first access to patients and want to help make decisions, while complying with the need for a faculty member to be appropriately involved and conceding to the patient's increased amount of control over decision making.

Link and Buchsbaum (1984, p. 494), who have made several comparisons of ambulatory and inpatient teaching, note that patients often seek ambulatory care for problems related to "loneliness, poverty, disturbing thoughts or fears, somatic effects of psychosocial conflict, validation of the self-perceived sick state, the need for information, or help with coping with various bureaucracies." This results in remarkable nonconcordance between physician and patient as to the nature of the problem. Physicians and patients have very different criteria for judging the nature of the problem, the appropriateness of treatments, and the desirability of outcomes. The predictive value of many tests is low due to the low prevalance of disease in ambulatory patient populations. Many problems are self-limited, such that symptomatic treatments have a high "cure" rate. Other differences described by Link and Buchsbaum are organized according to issues of time, the doctor-patient relationship, goals, and clinical decision making:

Time. Inpatient teaching can take as much time as necessary. The patient is at the mercy of hospital schedules, although only for a few days. Ambulatory teaching occurs in many brief "teachable" moments over long periods of time. Medical data therefore are gathered in-depth on the inpatient service but only selectively in ambulatory patients. This markedly changes the nature of the teaching discussions. Plans that result from such discussions may be implemented sequentially in outpatients, while done simultaneously in inpatients, resulting in another round of scheduled in-depth discussions that are not held for outpatients.

Doctor-Patient Relationship. The patient is remarkably passive in the hospital, is dependent on physical support systems, and is removed from the usual psychosocial support systems. The exact opposite is true for ambulatory patients. This shift of power causes the ambulatory student-physician to negotiate diagnoses and treatments carefully, with resultant implications for the teacher, who wishes to support the learner yet assure quality care. The degree to which the physician imposes certain decisions on the patient varies more in the ambulatory setting and depends considerably on "the patient's desires, cognitive capacity, emotional state, the severity of the disease, the efficacy of the proposed therapy, and the public health aspects of the case" (Luile & Buchsbaum 1984 pp. 497–498). Finally, patients judge ambulatory physician performance more overtly on behavioral, rather than technical, criteria. This has implications for how the teacher relates to the learner, who is relating to the patient. How does an experienced faculty physician care for a patient indirectly through the learner, yet transmit warmth and compassion that are somewhat less developed qualities in some learners?

Goals. "Cure" is much harder to define in some ambulatory situations than in inpatients whose discharge is synonomous with "cure," at least for that episode of care. Less dramatic goals of treatment, often not considered in inpatients, are control of symptoms, increases in function, and emotional reassurance. Preventive medicine and screening for disease are critical, although poorly defined, goals that require different types of discussions between teacher and learner than do traditional diagnostic and management plans.

Clinical Decision Making. Inpatient teaching is based on huge quantities of data, collected and confirmed by several members of an inpatient team. Ambulatory teaching is based on minimal data, always incomplete, collected by one learner and, perhaps, confirmed by the teacher. Uncertainty is rampant, and outcomes of decisions are often not known for a long time, if at all in the case of some preventive interventions. The teaching of clinical reasoning and decision making is difficult even with extensive data. In the face of uncertainty, teachers have to use more art than science to teach clinical reasoning. Scheduling problems may cause the learner to miss follow-up that does occur, and communication problems may subvert the educational value of ordering tests and making referrals.

Objectives

The description of ambulatory teaching activities and the comparison of inpatient and ambulatory teaching described in the preceding sections suggest that there are specific learning objectives peculiar to ambulatory teaching. For example, Schatz (1985) has described certain learning objectives that caused the redesign of an ambulatory internal medicine training program, which changed from a half-day per week throughout 3 years of residency training to a full-time assignment to an ambulatory practice and health care team that lasted several months. These are the learning objectives that caused this program change:

1. To evaluate new patients, and to follow them up as diagnostic and therapeutic maneuvers unfold;
2. To develop an ongoing relation with each patient so as to understand the psychosocial milieu in which the patient lives and works;
3. To be identified by the patient as his or her "doctor";
4. To supervise, as much as possible, the patient's care on a continuing basis and to understand the natural course of illness;
5. To participate actively in those management decisions that might require urgent or elective invasive tests or hospital admission.

An important study by McGlynn and associates (1978) described, through questionnaires and personal interviews, certain factors that contributed to optimal learning of ambulatory medicine by internal medicine residents. Characteristics of the practice that contributed to learning included the opportunity to follow patients over time, to examine and treat patients and thereby encounter many ambulatory problems or diseases, and to communicate and work directly with consultants and with faculty supervisors. Characteristics of practice that interfered with learning included inadequate numbers or types of patients, inadequate space or support staff, and inadequate time to see patients and receive supervision. Characteristics of the learner-patient relationship that contributed to learning included residents having opportunities to encounter, manage, and follow up patient problems; to establish strong relationships and rapport; to see clinical responses and perceive that treatments are beneficial; and to be able to adjust treatments and observe responses that correlate with changes in historical, examination, and laboratory parameters. McGlynn and associates concluded that successful ambulatory teaching rests on the creation of a series of feedback or cybernetic loops in which strong relationships are created between the resident physician, an adequate number and diversity of patients, and accessible and useful faculty or consultants. Learners are thus at the center of an educational and clinical decision-making system; they make assessments and decisions, seek assessment and modification of those decisions from teachers, implement the decisions, and then observe and assess the effect of the decisions. The loop then starts over again. This work suggests several appropriate learning objectives for learners in an ambulatory setting:

1. Ambulatory practice should be organized to encourage the establishment of strong relationships between the learner, the teacher, the patient, and the patient's community.
2. The learner should have maximum responsibility consistent with his knowledge and experience, for patient care.
3. Teacher-learner interactions, discussions, and didactic teaching should emphasize learning how to make clinical decisions with incomplete data and in complex psychosocial situations.

4. Teacher-learner interactions should focus on identifying learner deficiencies and weaknesses, establishing specific plans to remedy these deficiencies, and monitoring progress to help learners achieve competency.

Teaching Techniques

The learning objectives just described can be accomplished by using certain teaching techniques. As might be expected, these techniques have some overlap with techniques used in inpatient and bedside teaching, since there is considerable similarity in style and objectives of these clinical teaching formats. (The reader may wish to refer to some material in chapters 7 and 8 regarding characteristics of successful teachers, the teaching of clinical problem solving, and techniques of demonstrating and practicing procedures.) However, the application of these techniques to ambulatory teaching may be somewhat different than to inpatient teaching, and the discussion of techniques that follows will expand upon certain unique aspects of ambulatory teaching.

Adopt Characteristics of Excellent Ambulatory Clinical Teachers

Studies previously cited have described characteristics of excellent clinical teachers, as determined by learner evaluations. Certain unique characteristics distinguish superior teachers of ambulatory medicine, although physician teachers certainly can be exceptionally good in both inpatient and outpatient settings. Stritter and Baker (1982) have studied the preferences of family medicine residents to determine what constitutes outstanding ambulatory teaching. Their study was based on the following accepted principles of excellence in resident education (p. 34):

Residents and preceptors should agree that the content of teaching is important and related to desired future competencies;

The preceptor should set expectations or "contract" with the resident concerning the nature of the learning experience;

The preceptor should develop instruction and learning experiences that are well organized;

The preceptor must be aware of the power of the role model he provides and take advantage of it in his teaching;

The preceptor must be conscious of the art of his teaching, and relate well interpersonally with his residents;

The resident should be given specific responsibilities in patient care which make him an active participant in the learning process;

Well-designed and systematic feedback should be provided to the resident during and after the execution of his clinical responsibilities

Based on these principles, Stritter and Baker (1982) studied the characteristics of excellent family medicine preceptors in the two areas of content of resident clinical teaching and teaching behaviors. With regard to content areas (which may not apply to all areas of ambulatory or primary care teaching), residents rated the following five areas most strongly:

1. The use of patient management skills, including skills in the management of chronic disease;
2. The treatment of primary care problems, including the management of common acute adult medical problems;
3. The ability to take psychosocial issues into consideration, including interviewing and family dynamic skills;
4. The financial and business aspects of practice, including patient education and record keeping systems;

5. The understanding of disease, including pathophysiologic processes and laboratory parameters.

Teaching behaviors favored by residents were grouped into six factors. The excellent ambulatory preceptor is the physician who

1. Modeled the role of a family physician, including displaying confidence in the roles of both teacher and family physician;
2. Valued the learner as an individual, including being fair to each resident and being accessible for consultation;
3. Accepted the resident's role as learner but treated the resident as a colleague and was willing to scrutinize his own views when presented with new information or ideas;
4. Directed the resident's learning by identifying the problems or therapies he considered important and setting realistic goals and objectives;
5. Provided information by explaining the basis for actions and decisions and answering questions clearly and precisely;
6. Provided and asked for evaluation by correcting residents without belittling or demeaning them and giving positive feedback when deserved.

The importance of the preceptor as a role model is highlighted by Brownell and McDougall (1984, p. 856), who note, "The attending physician's behaviour at the bedside enables the trainees to learn about some of the broader aspects of medical care: responding to patient's fears and anxieties, dealing with the dying or dead patient, consoling the family, managing time effectively, cooperating with allied health care professionals and coping with the inevitable stress of the profession. The success of the attending physician in these areas will ultimately determine the extent to which the trainee will incorporate similar skills into his or her own professional performance."

Bibace and co-workers (1981) investigated four types of teaching styles adopted by ambulatory preceptors, also in family medicine. These four styles, adapted from a classification scheme of physician-patient relationships developed by Byrne and Long (1976), are *assertive, suggestive, collaborative,* and *facilitative.* No one style is appropriate for all situations in the office, and the excellent teacher adopts the most productive style depending on the learner's learning style. The assertive style includes giving directions, asking questions, giving information, and asking self-answering questions. The suggestive style is less directive and includes offering opinions, suggesting with questions or statements, and relating personal experiences. The collaborative style includes eliciting student ideas (and accepting at least some of them). Finally, the facilitative style is even more passive and includes offering feelings, encouragement, and using silence. The reader may recognize a similarity between this continuum and that described in chapter 4.

Finally, excellence in ambulatory precepting was studied in private physicians who provided preceptorships for medical students. MacDonald and Bass (1983) studied the characteristics of the physician and his practice that correlated with excellent evaluations by the students of the quality of teaching provided. Teachers were evaluated in six areas: breadth of knowledge, clarity of instruction, interpersonal interaction skills, friendliness, enthusiasm, and a global measure. The practice characteristics that correlated most closely with teaching excellence were group (vs. solo) practice, high referral rates to allied health professionals, the use of a problem-oriented medical record including medication lists, a higher volume of patients, larger number of exam rooms available for use, and the degree to which responsibility was delegated to the student. Taken together, these factors suggest that success in teaching in one's private office depends most on whether the physician-teacher spends enough time with the student, the volume of patients is high and widely diverse, the records are sufficiently well-organized to allow the student to become integrated into the patient's care for the short time of his rotation, and the student is allowed to become as involved and responsible as possible for the medical care rendered.

Base all Teacher-Learner Interactions on Negotiation and Contracting

Except when precluded by dire emergencies (of either a medical or scheduling nature), one of the critical aspects of ambulatory teaching is the opportunity to care for the patient indirectly through the learner by a process of negotiation and contracting. This model does not suggest that patients be abandoned to learners of variable ability and experience, but that the important cybernetic learning loops described by McGlynn and co-workers (1978) will not operate unless the learner and patient first establish a relationship, and then the learner and teacher establish a relationship, within which the outcome of the teacher-learner interaction will be negotiated. This differs somewhat from inpatient teaching where the choice of management plans is likely more limited, and the locus of responsibility for making decisions more clearly lies, at least ultimately, with the attending physician. Of critical importance in meeting the learning objectives of ambulatory teaching is the teacher's ability to allow the learner as much freedom as possible in caring for the patient and making decisions, without compromising medical care quality. Each teacher will have a different threshhold of quality at which his need to "take over and do it right" will become overwhelming. Using a model of negotiation and contracting will insure that the teacher can approach that threshhold gradually and comfortably, meanwhile building the confidence of the learner so that he can assume more responsibility, to the extent possible. The care provided by the learner will never be exactly the same as if provided by the teacher, but the teacher must allow differences, to the extent that differences of equal quality exist. The inability of the teacher to do this suggests that the teacher perhaps ought not to be teaching.

The model of negotiation and contracting consists of the following set of four steps (Hart & Kurtz 1983):

1. In the *precontracting* phase, the ambulatory teacher or preceptor meets with the learner for brief introductions and discussions. These are obviously more extensive for a resident beginning a 3-year longitudinal assignment than for a student starting a 1-month preceptorship. The learner learns of the necessary early stages of observation and assessment and that a more detailed contract (and hopefully one allowing increasing independence of action) will be negotiated after the observation period. The learner must agree to the observation and assessment period and to the setting of a contract at the end of that period.

2. In the *initial observation and feedback period* the teacher assigns various tasks and duties under supervision and makes an assessment of the learner's knowledge, attitudes, and skills. The teacher makes specific arrangements to discuss the learner's performance in some detail. This period may last only one or a few days for a student on a brief rotation, or an entire orientation month for a family practice resident. During this period, the learner must be comfortable in performing tasks, some of which will have been previously mastered, under supervision and in the unique style of the particular office. The content of a complete physical examination is much the same anywhere, but the routines are different in every office. In addition to teacher assessments of learner performance, the learner will make self-assessments and be prepared to discuss these self-assessments with the teacher in a nonthreatening and mature fashion (which will depend considerably on the style and the interpersonal skills of the teacher).

3. The *contracting* phase is when the actual objectives for the experience are determined. These objectives should be specific and include a negotiation of how the learner will function, how learning will progress, and how and when feedback will occur. The learner must take an active role in this negotiating and contracting phase, or the contract will be more like an authoritarian directive, which the learner

may or may not accept. A part of this active learner role is for the learner to request assessment and feedback upon his completion of the negotiated activities.

4. In the final phase, *implementation of instruction and assessment*, the teacher arranges appropriate experiences and activities that will allow the learner to achieve the objectives. These activities may be as disparate as accompanying the teacher to a nursing home or on a home visit, experiencing the office in the role of a patient, being assigned for an entire residency to a health care team caring for several thousand patients, or using various special outpatient training modalities such as simulated or trained patients. During these activities, the teacher provides both instruction and supervision by acting as a role model, by providing specific teaching in content areas or providing for the teaching through other teachers (e.g., partners, nursing staff, or physicians in other specialties or offices), and by continually assessing learner performance and giving feedback to the learner. Again, that assessment may be as brief as a few occasional words to a student spending a half-day per week in the physician's office, or as extensive as quarterly evaluation and feedback sessions for primary care residents. During this phase, the learner will benefit by being as active as possible in requesting instruction, references, or outside resources and activities. The time pressures of ambulatory medicine sometimes take precedence in the teacher's thinking unless reminded of educational priorities by their beneficiary (the learner). The learner should, of course, indicate a receptivity to receiving feedback, but the teacher should be receptive to feedback as well. The true cybernetic learning loop of assessment, instruction, and feedback includes students giving feedback to teachers.

Margon (1979) describes the characteristics of negotiating a contract with ambulatory care residents who will be training over a three-year period. The teacher may, for instance, relate a number of past experiences with precepting to indicate the possible forms a contract might take and to indicate what has worked well for that particular teacher. This technique also shows what teacher's needs might require more careful negotiation with the needs of the learner. Many outpatient teachers, for example, feel that they must know everything to be seen as competent by learners. This is not only unrealistic but unnecessary. A clear statement of the teacher's strengths and weaknesses will help clarify this situation to residents.

Written self-assessments of resident abilities are particularly helpful, such as a list of outpatient procedures that the learner can and cannot do competently. Specific areas of content weakness might be assessed by formal cognitive testing. Residents also prefer negotiating the specific style of instruction and supervision, such as having the teacher observe the resident with patients randomly, or being available for more formal consultations as determined by the residents (which is appropriate for more experienced residents). Despite the open-ended nature of these agreements, a certain number of conferences, patient discussions, chart reviews, direct observations, or videotape sessions should be specified so as to satisfy the teacher's responsibilities. Some residents, for instance, will avoid certain types of experiences or teacher interactions because of discomfort or feelings of inadequacies. This is far more likely to happen in the less structured environment of the office, as opposed to the hospital. The teacher may have to make very specific arrangements to observe the resident directly, for example, since that is an experience that a teacher may value but a resident may not. Finally, the timing and method of giving feedback must be specifically negotiated. Some residents prefer a certain time, such as immediately after leaving the examination room, while others can benefit from and cope with feedback being given while the teacher, learner, and patient are still together.

This contracting method of teaching in the ambulatory setting is important for several reasons, not the least of which is that there are often wide discrepancies between goals of teachers and learners. For example, London and Green (1977) studied the content goals of family medicine residents, family medicine faculty, and volunteer subspecialty faculty in a family medicine residency program. There was little disagreement between residents and family medicine faculty in whether certain problems or procedures should be learned by residents, but there was great discrepancy in all specialties between subspecialists and residents. A resident rotation in a subspecialty with a teacher who has markedly different ideas than the resident about what should be learned would be an educational disaster without proper negotiation and contracting (and may even be a problem after the negotiation).

Negotiation also is helpful for reducing differences in style and educational process. When family medicine residents and faculty were offered choices, such as "to discuss therapeutic plan," "to discuss diagnostic plan," "to discuss differential diagnosis," "to discuss patient education plan," "to verify a physical finding," or "to obtain information concerning medication" as possible options in a resident-faculty interaction, Tibbles (1985) found disagreement between teacher and resident in about 50% of interactions. In circumstances of time pressure, as Tibbles (p. 15) notes, "the greatest perceived need by the supervisor is the one most likely met." This priority is not likely to result in a productive learning experience for the resident.

This negotiating and contracting approach can be incorporated into a more extensive problem-solving precepting method. Esposito and colleagues (1983) have described a precepting method that focuses entirely on the teacher-resident interaction and the problem solving that the teacher can do in that interaction. The teacher begins by identifying initial impressions, gathering data to confirm or refute those impressions, identifying problems displayed by the resident during the interaction, developing teaching goals, devising methods to achieve goals, and evaluating the outcome of the teaching. For example, as a resident presents a case for discussion, the teacher may conclude that the resident is ignoring a highly likely diagnosis in the differential. The teacher could then question the resident further about that diagnosis or interview and exam the patient directly, conclude that the resident is indeed missing the likely diagnosis, negotiate with the resident the exploration of that diagnosis as a possibility, find specific references for the resident to study, provide brief didactic summaries, ask the resident to interview and exam the patient further in light of the new information, and evaluate the resident's decisions in light of the new information. Of course, in ambulatory teaching, this process may have to be accomplished in only a few minutes. Therein lies the challenge!

Use Assessment, Instruction and Evaluation, and Feedback to Close the Cybernetic Teaching Loop

Ambulatory teaching is a more personal, one-on-one teaching relationship than other forms of teaching. Whether the teacher is in a hospital-based ambulatory facility or in a private office, whether the learner is a student on a 1-month preceptorship or a resident on a 3-year model health center assignment, the interaction is between one teacher and one learner concerning the care of one patient. This one-on-one communication led Whitman and Schwenk (1984) to adapt a model of communication known as the Johari Window to clinical teaching, so as to better define the role and activities of the ambulatory teacher. From this adaptation, four types of knowledge, attitudes, and skills can be described:

1. Shared knowledge, attitudes, and skills (KAS) are those domains of learning possessed by the learner and of which the teacher is aware. A student may know how to start an intravenous line, and the teacher knows that the student knows how.

2. Hidden KAS are those domains possessed by the learner, but not known by the teacher. The teacher may not know that the student also knows how to draw arterial blood gases.

3. Known needs are those aspects of KAS not possessed by the learner, but the teacher is aware of these deficiencies. The teacher may know that the learner does not know how to place a permanent arterial cannula.

4. Unknown needs are those aspects of clinical KAS not possessed

by the learner, and the teacher is not aware of these deficiencies. The learner does not know of the Swan-Ganz catheter for measuring central hemodynamic parameters, and the teacher does not realize the learner is unaware of this.

This description of specific types of learning needs suggests an agenda for ambulatory teachers. The first function of the teacher is to uncover some of the hidden KAS through assessment, so that the teacher will become aware of some of the learning needs of the learner. The second function of the teacher is to increase the shared KAS category by reducing the size of the known needs category. This occurs through instruction. The third function is to link assessment and instruction through feedback and evaluation. Specific techniques for these functions follow.

Assessment. Assessment of learner KAS occurs through questioning (knowledge), developing professional intimacy (attitudes), and observing (skills). The use of both closed and open questions is useful for assessing knowledge. Closed questions have a small range of possible correct answers; open questions allow for a wide range of appropriate responses. Usually, it is good to begin the assessment of a learner's knowledge with an open question such as, "What are your impressions of the patient's problem?" More closed questions can be used to understand the learner's knowledge more specifically, with a return to more open questions to uncover more hidden knowledge and needs. Questioning does not mean interrogating. Learners need to understand that the purpose of questioning is to help the teacher to target instruction, not to belittle them. Self-assessment questioning is an equally valuable technique, "What have we just discussed that you have not previously studied?" Questions can be factual, or more broadening, justifying, or hypothetical.

The assessment of learner attitudes is really an assessment of their budding professional behaviors. The teacher can really only know a learner's attitudes by his behavior. The assessment of professional attitudes and behaviors is quite analogous to the assessment of patient health care beliefs and health care seeking behaviors, which is something that physician-teachers do regularly. There are four ways that teachers can behave that will encourage learners to reveal their attitudes accurately and comfortably. First, the teacher can develop rapport by sharing personal thoughts, opinions, and stories in an open and self-aware way that makes clear that self-disclosure and personal vulnerability are valued. Inclusion of the learner in personal, family and social activities is particularly helpful. Second, the teacher can show genuine interest in the learner by including him as a full participant in office and professional activities, such as staff meetings. Third, the teacher can be accessible by being patient with the learner's presence and ideas, making clear when the teacher is willing to discuss problems (medical or otherwise), and recognizing the extra work required to be useful to learners. Fourth, the teacher can be empathetic and nonjudgemental by remembering the many fears, anxieties, and uncertainties of medical education; by responding with compassion; and by acknowledging the general value of a learner's ideas without implying that all are correct. These four behaviors will encourage the learner to express himself clearly and reveal attitudes accurately and without distortion.

Observation is a critical assessment skill, just as it is a critical clinical skill (Engel 1965). Observation requires standards or criteria, so the teacher may wish to develop checklists for common procedures performed in the office. Breaking a skill into specific steps reduces the likelihood of errors and omissions. When observing a learner, nonverbal cues may be significant: How comfortable and confident did the learner seem? Did the learner tremble, seem disorganized, or show irritation to cover up uncertainty? Feedback from patients, nursing, and office staff is very helpful; however, direct observation by the teacher while the learner performs a clinical skill, is most important. As noted by Eichna (1975, p. 731), "Clinical skills are no longer actively taught. A casual pass is made in the course on physical diagnosis, but students are not observed talking to patients or examining them. We are training future physicians who have never been observed to elicit a history or take a physical examination—not in the second year physical diagnosis course, not in third year clinical clerkships, and not during house officership." Wray and Friedland (1983) confirm that the problem described by Eichna continues.

To remedy the problem described by Eichna, several imaginative and innovative techniques that were developed recently can be used to obtain feedback from patients:

The use of actors and actresses trained to simulate patients (Callaway et al. 1977);

The use of actual patients with various diseases trained to report on their medical care experiences (Stillman et al. 1980);

The use of various manikins and other mechanical simulators such as "Harvey," which is used for assessing and teaching heart auscultation skills (Penta & Kofman 1973);

The use of two-way mirrors and videotape to allow direct observation of learner-patient interaction without disturbing the learner-patient relationship (Cassata et al. 1977);

Direct observation techniques such as "intensive precepting" used in some residency training programs (Demers 1978).

Actors or trained patients can be used to assess and evaluate the learner's abilities in interview or physical examination skills; for example, patient education skills can be accurately assessed with patients trained in noting characteristics used by physicians that are known to promote successful patient learning (Callaway et al. 1977). These patients can report on whether certain questions were asked, the manner and demeanor of the learner, and whether certain physical examination techniques were performed and if done correctly. Some studies (Stillman et al. 1980) have obtained permission from residents in advance to schedule these "patients" as part of a regular office schedule so that the resident has no knowledge that a particular patient is part of such an exercise. This is about as realistic an assessment of certain ambulatory patient care skills as could be made. Another equally realistic assessment technique is the use of mirrors and videotape, although more time for debriefing is required. Reviewing videotapes with a small group of residents or students is particularly effective. Each learner contributes one videotaped patient interaction for small group discussion (see chapter 6) for self- and peer-review, which is a powerful assessment and instructional tool. Finally, direct observation, although very time consuming, is also very useful. The teacher can merely introduce himself as a colleague assisting the learner, and observe the interview and exam quietly from a corner of the exam room. The seeming artificiality disappears rapidly, and the data gathered during this type of assessment are valuable in their accuracy and immediacy.

Instruction. The instruction of KAS requires the teacher to use the techniques of sharing experience (knowledge), role modeling (attitudes), and demonstration and practice (skills). The ways that the teacher instructs depend upon how relatively active or passive the teacher wishes to be. The active teacher will share "war stories," or the accumulated wisdom of years of practice. Describing difficult cases from the past, current diagnostic dilemmas, and cases that were either triumphs or failures is particularly helpful. The teacher who wishes to be less active and wants the learner to be relatively more so can use more open-ended techniques such as brainstorming, open-ended questioning, challenging and summarizing. The purpose of brainstorming is to generate differential diagnoses or multiple therapeutic options. Not all options have to be correct, but all are worth discussing. The teacher can pose hypothetical cases or situations to the learner, or ask about hypothetical variations of a current case. "If the age of this patient with rectal bleeding were 20 instead of 60 years, how would it change your approach?" The use of questioning as an instructing technique requires that the questions be open-ended, such that the learner is required to clarify, correlate, critique, evaluate, analyze, interpret, and predict, rather than answer yes or no. Learners should also be challenged by being asked to support, justify, and defend their ideas, but this requires a larger measure of rapport and skills in constructive confrontation. Asking students to summarize is less threatening if the teacher always summarizes his ideas and suggestions about a problem as a way of achieving the goal of transmitting facts. Finally, learners should be particularly active at times, by being assigned responsibility for preparing lectures, making minireports on questions that arise in the course of regular patient care, or completing more major educational and research projects. Some preceptorships have prepared reading lists pertinent to their specialty that are assigned, along with projects requiring further independent study (Flaherty 1983).

The instruction of attitudes through role modeling is difficult because it suggests that certain norms exist. Interestingly, certain characteristics do appear consistently in the literature on successful patient care behaviors for physicians. The characteristics are remarkably similar to the characteristics of ideal clinical teachers (Stritter et al. 1975; Irby 1978; Lamkin et al. 1983). These are the ways that ambulatory teachers can be, and the behaviors they may want their learners to emulate: *capable, sensitive, enthusiastic,* and *genuine.*

McDermott (1982) noted that the "deep belief in the necessity of thoroughness is the most important element of medical education." The teacher can provide excellent medical care, be organized in both patient care and teaching responsibilities, be current and well-read, and explain the basis for decisions as ways of demonstrating capability.

The easiest way to teach sensitivity to the needs of patients is for the teacher to be sensitive to the needs of the learner, the Golden Rule for medical teachers described in chapter 8. By being empathetic to the anxieties and fears of medical learners and being patient and compassionate about their failures and inadequacies, the teacher models an appropriate way to treat both patients and learners. The teacher can demonstrate enthusiasm by being accessible and available to learners, interested in their problems and needs, and dynamic and energetic in planning and implementing teaching activities. Finally, the teacher can be genuine by being willing to demonstrate and defend the way he teaches and provides patient care; by being explicit and honest about his own uncertainties, difficulties, and ambiguities; and by being willing to say, "I don't know."

Instruction of skills through demonstration and practice follows the old surgical dictum, "See one, do one, teach one," with the added insurance of, "Do one more" before proceeding to teaching. These techniques are well-described in chapter 8 on bedside teaching and apply equally well whether the "bed" is located in a hospital or office.

Feedback and Evaluation. Feedback connects assessment and instruction. When students and residents are assessed, information about their performance needs to be given back to them so that they know what they did well and what needs to be improved. Thus, giving feedback is a form of instruction. In order to encourage learners to be more revealing and self-critical, thus making future assessment easier, teachers should give feedback that is

As specific as possible;
Positive only when deserved;
Not demeaning when critical;
Understandable;
About things that can be changed;
Well timed.

In addition, recommendations of the Family Practice Faculty Development Center of Texas (Williams 1980) are helpful. Feedback should be based on systematic observation, should emphasize change in behavior and progress toward a goal, should be paraphrased by the learner to see if it is understood, should be conducted in an unhurried and comfortable atmosphere, and should allow the person being evaluated to provide input. With regard to summative evaluation, the dreaded evaluation form that often accompanies learners in any setting, the suggestion of the Clinical Evaluation Project of the Association of American Medical Colleges (1984) that psychometric solutions are not substitutes for the judgements of the teacher is most pertinent. Evaluation is a natural outcome of the cycle of assessment, feedback, and instruction, and the teacher is the best person to make specific comments and judgments about the cognitive, attitudinal, and psychomotor skills of the learner. Much of the discomfort teachers feel about evaluation can be alleviated by adopting this attitude: The teacher always tells the learner anything that is written down, and anything worth telling the learner is worth writing down.

Tips

1. Orientation is a critical first step in any ambulatory teaching experience. The length and intensity may be different for a third-year student on preceptorship than for a resident beginning three years of family practice training, but the principle is the same: Pretend the learner is a new partner or faculty member. What would he need to know to function effectively for one day in the office? Walking through the routine of one patient encounter is helpful. Having the learner be a patient—starting with making an appointment over telephone and ending with a trip to the laboratory, with filling out forms in between—is even more instructive.

2. Introducing students to patients is always difficult. Is the student a "trainee", a "student", a "smart young man from the medical school", or a "doctor"? Is he "working for me for awhile," "just watching me today," "getting some extra experience," or (chuckle, chuckle) "checking to see if I'm doing a good job"? Introducing a student as a "student doctor" who is "working with me for a month" is probably most accurate, least deceptive to the patient, and least demeaning to the student.

3. Introducing a teacher to patients cared for by residents, when the teacher is consulted or wishes to intensively precept and observe,

is sometimes cumbersome or embarrassing. The teacher can simply introduce himself as a colleague who is assisting the resident, much like a staff physician who might consult a colleague regarding a difficult or interesting problem. The patient often becomes aware of the learning status of the resident but is usually flattered with the extra attention rather than annoyed.

4. A critical determinant of the educational value of an ambulatory experience for either student or resident is the attitude of the office personnel. This may not be a problem in a university outpatient clinic, but is a frequent issue in private offices. Usually, however, the office staff will take their lead from the physician teacher, who must be particularly clear about the value of the educational experience, without compromising quality patient care. This is often a subconscious fear of the office personnel (and perhaps the physician teacher), and more so in the ambulatory setting where the physician-patient relationship is more sensitive, and the "checks and balances" of inpatient education are not present.

5. Maintaining patient schedules and flow is critical. These can be severely disrupted with a third- or fourth-year student in the office. A useful strategy is to assign the student to take a complete history on a patient requesting a complete physical exam, or a patient presenting for chronic disease follow-up, during which time the physician-teacher can care for several other patients alone. Both educational and patient care needs are met with this strategy.

6. A generally accepted wisdom amongst ambulatory teachers is that learners of various levels take or save time in the teaching-patient care trade-off in the following order (ranked from those learners that require more guidance and cost the most time, to those learners who save time because they provide more independent patient care or require less direct supervision for their level of responsibility

Third-year medical students;
Fourth-year medical students;
First-year residents (interns);
Preclinical (first- and second-year) students;

Second-year residents;
Third-year residents.

For example, a first-year student and a third-year resident can be handled comfortably in a small office. A third-year student and an intern together might be a logistical disaster.

7. Since the establishment of a strong learner-patient relationship is probably the strongest predictor of the educational value of ambulatory teaching, any techniques that further this process are worthwhile. These may include posting the learner's name visibly in the office, printing business/appointment cards for residents, having the receptionist or nurse use the learner's name frequently with the patient (in a positive context), having the teacher introduced as a colleague rather than a supervisor, making frequent reference to the diagnosis and plan generated by the learner ("I think Student Doctor Smith is correct about the need for a chest x-ray to investigate your cough."), and supporting follow-up by the patient with the learner.

Conclusion

Ambulatory teaching is simultaneously one of the most important parts of medical education and one of the hardest types of teaching to do. Certain unique aspects of patient care logistics and patient expectations make the usual traditions of inpatient teaching inapplicable. The interplay between patient care and educational priorities and objectives is dynamic and sensitive and requires particular skill by the physician teacher to manage such a fragile balance. The dominant principle is that the strength of the learner-patient relationship is the best predictor of the impact of ambulatory teaching. The teacher-learner relationship must be constructed to enhance, rather than detract from, the learner-patient relationship. Specific teacher behaviors and specific skills in assessment, instruction, and feedback and evaluation can then be applied to make the learner-patient relationship have simultaneous educational and patient care value.

EPILOGUE

Connoisseurship and Creativity in Teaching

Thus far, we have addressed our readers in the third person, e.g., "physician teachers should . . ." In this last chapter, we would like to address you more personally in the second person. Because we have known and worked with many medical teachers, we feel we know you, the unseen reader, in a very personal way. We hope that, by reading thus far, you have a personal sense of who we are and what our aims are. Ultimately, we have two aims: to help you become *connoisseurs* of teaching and to become more *creative* teachers.

What do we mean by becoming a "connoisseur" of teaching? Basically, a connoisseur is a person with informed and astute discrimination, especially concerning the arts or matters of taste. Eliot Eisner, who began his academic career in art education and today teaches at the Stanford University School of Education, has been the most noteworthy proponent of the "connoisseur of teaching" concept. According to Eisner (1979) a connoisseur is someone who knows how to look, see, and appreciate. Thus, educational connoisseurship is the art of knowing and appreciating what is educationally significant.

To become a connoisseur of anything requires experience. As

Eisner points out, to become a connoisseur of wine, one must drink a great deal of it. Frank Prial (1984, p. 103), the wine editor for *The New York Times,* recommends a basic course on wine but also says, "Just bear in mind the old adage: There is no substitute for opening bottles."

Of course, if only experience were needed, who would not be an educational connoisseur? If experience were the only requirement, all of you would by now be connoisseurs of clinical teaching, based on the thousands of hours of lectures, morning reports, work rounds, and grand rounds you have attended as a medical student, resident, and staff physician.

The catch is that to be a connoisseur one must *see as well as look.* An educational connoisseur is someone who can see what is subtle, complex, and important in the teaching-learning process, and this requires *knowledge* about teaching and learning. In fact, the word "connoisseur" is derived from the Latin, *cognoscere,* to get acquainted with or to know thoroughly. The word "connoisseur" thus shares the same Latin root as the word "cognition." The need for knowledge, as well as experience, was highlighted in a *New York Times* article on antiques. In an article about Charles Santore, a man who began collecting Windsor chairs twenty years ago and now has written a book about these chairs, the antique editor, Rita Rief (1983, p. 36), commented, "Today Mr. Santore relies upon his own educated eye, a great deal of acquired knowledge, and common sense to identify the Windsor designs he encounters."

Based on our personal and professional relationships with many clinicians, we feel confident that you have common sense and can develop an educated eye. We hope that this book has added to your knowledge of teaching and learning so that you will feel equipped to become an educational connoisseur. The benefit to you of being a connoisseur of teaching is that you will be able to learn about teaching in every educational encounter, even when someone else is teaching. As an educational connoisseur, you will be able to see what works and what does not. What helps students learn? What teaching format is best for a particular educational objective? What is the educational objective of this session? How will the teacher know if it is accomplished? Educational connoisseurs have the advantage of creating their own personal data base on the teaching profession. Once you are a connoisseur, the knowledge you will gain regarding clinical teaching will be even greater and more personally relevant than the knowledge we have tried to impart in this book.

How do you develop an astute eye? The answer lies in being systematic in your observation of teaching done by you and others. For example, Dr. Jerome P. Kassirer (1983) of Tufts-New England Medical Center had observed that case presentations were boring for teachers and students. Dr. Kassirer, whom we would consider a connoisseur of teaching, developed his own approach to the teaching of diagnostic reasoning based on the hypothesis-driven interative method that physicians actually use in clinical practice. In his conferences, the student does not present the case (Kassirer points out that patients do not "present their case" to the doctor); rather the student is the source of all the patient's clinical data but provides information only when asked. The learners and the teacher may ask any questions they wish, but anyone asking a question must first justify it. Participants are asked what diagnostic hypotheses they had in mind and why they asked the question. When questions are answered, participants are asked what they learned and how the information refined or changed their hypotheses.

Although he has not proposed a plan to formally evaluate his approach to teaching clinical medicine by iterative hypothsis testing, Kassirer feels comfortable with it because he knows that it is based on sound theories of human problem-solving and on extensive observations of physicians solving real clinical problems. Moreover, it is greeted enthusiastically by participants who ask for additional sessions. In our view, Dr. Kassirer clearly uses his own educated eye, a great deal of acquired knowledge, and common sense to teach clinical problem-solving just as Mr. Santore does to identify the Windsor chairs he collects. Also, he compares his teaching sessions to traditional case presentations, just as Mr. Prial compares with past bottles every bottle of wine he opens.

To help you become more systematic in your comparisons and assessments, we can offer a set of questions you can ask when you teach and when you observe the teaching of colleagues. These questions were used by Reichsman and colleagues (1964) over twenty years ago when they systematically observed "undergraduate clinical teaching in action."

1. Did the attending physician and students see the patient together during or following the case presentation?
2. Were the students' techniques of interviewing and physical examination observed by staff members?
3. Were the primary data obtained by students evaluated by staff members as to accuracy and appropriate completeness?
4. Were correlations between medicine and basic sciences a part of the teaching sessions?
5. Was information about clinical syndromes and concepts taught in a clear manner?
6. Did the data of the case presentation form the basis for discussion of diagnosis and differential diagnosis?
7. Did the amount of information taught seem appropriate to the type and objective of the teaching sessions?

We must warn you. There is one serious side effect of becoming an educational connoisseur—you will be less tolerant of mediocre teaching. The same is true for wine. For those of us who are not connoisseurs of wine, cheap wine can be very enjoyable, but the wine connoisseur cannot enjoy it. Of course, when a wine is wonderful, the connoisseur perhaps savors it more than the rest of us. So, be aware that, as an educational connoisseur, excellent teaching will excite you more than it does the students, and poor teaching will leave you more frustrated.

Our second hope is that, in addition to becoming a connoisseur of teaching, you will become a more creative teacher. What do we mean by becoming a "creative" teacher? Basically, creativity is any activity that results in contributions to human experience that are _novel_ and _useful_ (Fig. E.1). Being novel in teaching means using good communication skills and being inventive with teaching techniques so that what students learn is memorable and meaningful. Being useful in teaching means that what is learned is correct, up-to-date, and relevant. It also means that students learn the process of problem solving and develop patient care attitudes that are appropriate for the medical profession.

In our experience, medical teachers who are novel, but not useful, are _charlatans_. Because students do not yet know medicine, they can be fooled into thinking that charlatans are great teachers. Perhaps you had such a teacher as a student or you know of one now. Medical

	Useful	Not useful
Novel	Creative teacher	Charlatan
Not novel	Pedantic bore	Old goat

FIG. E.1. Creative Teaching

school faculty often are thinking of such teachers when they accuse educational specialists of advocating that faculty should "entertain" students. We do not advocate only entertainment, nor defend charlatans. However, we also do not defend the opposite—the *pendantic bore* who is useful, but not novel—and neither should you!

No one dares defend the teacher who is neither useful nor novel. In fact, until recently, we could not even find a name for this combination (although some workshop participants have suggested "administrator" or "tenured faculty.") Finally we came across a murder mystery by Robert Barnard, *Death of an Old Goat* (1977). Professor Belville-Smith had bored university audiences in England with the same lecture for 50 years. Now he was crossing the Australian continent, doing precisely the same. Never before had the reaction been so extreme, however, for shortly after an undistinguished appearance at Drummondale University, the doddering old professor is found brutally murdered.

Physician teachers who are pedantic are "academic" in the pejorative sense of being scholarly to the point of being unaware of the real world. Perhaps because of subspecialization of the biomedical sciences, the language of many medical presentations may appear alien to the learners and the content abstract. A creative solution lies in the "metaphorical technique" (Best 1984, p. 166):

> The word metaphor comes from a Greek word that means to transfer. A metaphor transfers meaning; it extends, stretches, twists the meaning of words so that they apply to other objects, actions, or situations than those to which they originally applied. By the metaphorical technique I mean metaphor in its broadest, most inclusive sense. I include simile, allegory, analogy, parable, anecdote, fable, song. I mean *anything* that transfers and translates the abstract into the concrete, thus making the abstract more accessible and memorable.

The metaphor is well-suited to help medical teachers attract and maintain attention, promote thinking, and make what was learned memorable. In a survey of award-winning medical teachers, Whitman and Ferrey (1986) asked for examples of the metaphorical technique. We share some of these to encourage you to borrow, adopt, and develop your own.

Bursae function to reduce friction is like holding a partially filled balloon whose lining is coated with oil between your two palms and moving it back and forth. There is no wear and tear on the skin of your palms.

A cytotoxic T-cell is a "mafia" cell. In contact with a foreign or virus-infected cell, it gives the "kiss of death."

Interferon is a molecular "Paul Revere" that alerts cells that a "virus is coming."

To illustrate the effectiveness of surface tension produced by pleural fluid in keeping visceral pleura applied to the pariental pleura during respiration, ask a student to pull apart two wet glass sheets.

The personal physician thinks about the "numerators" of life and the epidemiologist the "numerators and denominators."

An ocular melanoma is shaped like a mushroom.

Creative teachers are *both* novel and useful. They reveal the "inner relevance" of what they teach (Kestin 1970). They are selective in their teaching methodologies and pay attention to their delivery skills and devices (Peitzman 1983). What they teach often does not appear in a textbook (Whitman, 1982). Can *you* become more creative? Research in the field of creativity suggests that when people are asked *to pretend* to be creative, they in fact *are* more creative. Stein's (1974) explanation of this tested phenomenon is that, through much of their lives, people are told that they are not creative and they proceed to validate this statement by not being creative. However, when people are perceived as being creative, they change into being more creative individuals by actualizing the creative potential that was there all along.

What can you do to become more creative? The steps laid down by Wallas (1926) to describe creative thinking can be applied to creative teaching: preparation, incubation, illumination, and verification. In other words, during the *preparation stage,* the creative teacher investigates the teaching assignment: "What impact do I want to have on students, i.e., what do I want students to know, value, and/or do as a result of my teaching?" During the *incubation stage,* the creative teacher is not devoting conscious thought to the teaching assignment, but work still continues on the subconscious level. When you are doing this subconscious work, mulling over your teaching assignments, you may sometimes get an "aha" feeling. During the *illumination stage,* the creative teacher becomes aware of how the topic can be presented. It is here that the organization of the content comes together with the process of presenting it. Finally, in the *verification stage,* the teacher teaches and the validity of the instruction is tested: "Did I have the desired impact on students?" Creativity, then, can be conceived as a process rather than a product (Whiting 1958; Stein 1974).

According to Papper (1984), a "creative clinician" is one who has great knowledge and experience, fine clinical judgment, the wisdom to know when conventional thinking is right or wrong, insight to seek options, and imagination to find them. Our experience tells us that many of you in the field of medical teaching, whether full-time, part-time, or voluntary, are these creative clinicians. Can you teach your residents and medical students to become so? Maybe. Papper thinks it is doubtful whether one can be directly taught to be a creative clinician. But, we feel strongly (as does Papper) that it is well worth the effort because it will awaken and free those who are unknowingly creative and it will challenge all teachers and learners to do their best and struggle towards this ideal. We may be surprised by unexpected progress. Perhaps the behavior most likely to predict success in this effort at teaching students to become creative clinicians is consistency. Whether you are in the classroom or in the clinical setting, what you *say* and what you *do* need to be consistent. If you treat your residents and students as you would have them treat their patients, you will free them to do their best.

In conclusion, we view clinical teaching as a form of communication. Since you already have highly developed communication skills, especially with regard to patients, we see you as a potentially excellent teacher. By becoming a connoisseur of teaching and giving yourself permission to be more creative, we predict that excellent teaching lies ahead for you. In fact, your best teaching has yet to occur, as is true for the best art work of an artist who won first place in an art fair. When the judge gave her the prize, she said, "You know, I didn't submit my best work!" The judge was surprised by that statement and asked her, "Why not?" She responded, "Because I haven't done it yet!" None of us have done our best teaching . . . yet.

Bibliography

Altman LK: The doctor's world: Med schools under attack. *Times* June 22:21, 1982.

Aspy DN, Roebuck FN: *Kids Don't Learn from People They Don't Like.* Amherst, MA, Human Resource Development Press, 1977.

Assoc Amer Med Colleges: The general professional education of the physician report (the GPEP Report). *J Med Educ* (Part 2) 59: 1–31, 1984.

Auden WH, Kronenberger J: *The Viking Book of Aphorisms.* Kingsport, TN, Penguin Books, 1981.

Barnard R: *Death of an Old Goat* New York: Walker & Co. 1977.

Barnes-McConnell PW: Leading discussions. In Ohmer M (ed): *On College Teaching.* San Francisco, Jossey-Bass Publishers, 1980. pp 62–100.

Barrows HS, Tamblyn RM: *Problem Based Learning: An Approach to Medical Education.* New York, Springer, 1980.

Beasley JW: Using private practice settings for academically intensive family practice clerkships. *J Fam Pract* 17: 877–882, 1983.

Becker RM, Stillman PL: A community-based pediatrics rotation for medical students. *Ariz Med* 37: 774–776, 1981.

Berquist WH, Phillips SR: *A Handbook for Faculty Development.* Washington, DC, Council for the Advancement of Small Colleges, 1975.

Bertakis KD: The communication of information from physician to patient: A method for increasing patient retention and satisfaction. *J Fam Pract* 5: 217–222, 1977.

Best JA: Teaching political theory: Meaning through metaphor. *Impr Coll Univ Teaching* 32: 165–168, 1984.

Bibace R, Catlin RJO, Quirk ME, Beattie KA, Slabaugh RC: Teaching styles in the faculty-resident relationship. *J Fam Pract* 13: 895–900, 1981.

Black D: *Medicine Man: A Young Doctor on the Brink of the 21st Century.* New York, Watts, 1985.

Blanchard K, Johnson S: *The One-Minute Manager.* New York, William Morrow & Co, 1982.

Bloom B et al.: *Taxonomy of Educational Objectives: Handbook I. Cognitive Domain.* New York, David McKay Co, 1956.

Blumenthal DA, McNeal-Steele MS, Bullard LL, Daniel SL, Satcher D: Introducing preclinical students to primary care through a community preceptorship program. *J Med Educ* 58: 179–185, 1983.

Bradford LP: The teaching-learning transaction. *Adult Educ* 8: 135–145, 1958.

Braughman MD: *Braughman's Handbook of Humor in Education.* West Nyack, NY, Parker, 1974.

Brookfield S: Discussion as an effective educational method. In Rosenblum SH (ed): *Involving Adults in the Educational Process,* no. 26, June, 1985.

Brownell AKW, McDougall GM: The patient as the focus of teaching. *Can Med Assoc J* 131: 855–857, 1984.

Byrne PS, Long BE: *Doctors Talking to Patients* London: Her Majesty's Stationery Office, 1976.

Callaway S, Bosshart DA, O'Donell AA: Patient simulators in teaching patient education skills to family practice residents. *J Fam Pract* 4: 709–712, 1977.

Caplan RM: Preceptorships in primary care: University of Iowa experience. *J Iowa Med Soc* 65: 143–147, 1975.

Casciato DA, Goldberg GA, May LA: Introduction of ambulatory medical training in a Veterans Administration hospital. *J Med Educ* 54: 484–490, 1979.

Cassata DM, Conroe RM, Clements PW: A program for enhancing medical interviewing using video-tape feedback in the family practice residency. *J Fam Pract* 4: 673–677, 1977.

Change Magazine: Guide to Effective Teaching. New York: Change Magazine Press, 1978.

Charney E: Internal medicine and pediatric residency education for primary care. *J Med Educ* 50 (Part 2): 129–136, 1975.

Christian HA: Osler: Recollections of an undergraduate medical student at John Hopkins. *Arch Intern Med* 84: 77–83, 1949.

Collins GF, Cassie JM, Daggett CJ: The role of the attending physician in clinical teaching. *J Med Educ* 53: 429–431, 1978.

Crow HE, Rohrer MM, Carley WC, Radke KF, Holden DM, Smith GF: Non-rotational teaching of obstetrics in a family practice residency. *J Fam Pract* 10: 831–834, 1980.

Darley W, Turner E: Leadership in curriculum planning. *J Assoc Am Med Coll* 25: 17, 1950.

Davis RH, Alexander LT: *The Lecture Method.* East Lansing, Michigan State University, 1977.

DeMers JL: Observational assessment of performance. In Morgan MK, Irby DM (eds.): *Evaluating Clinical Competence in the Health Professions.* St. Louis, C. V. Mosby, 1978.

Dittman A: Kinestic research and therapeutic processes: Further discussion. In Knapp PN (ed): *Expression of Emotions in Man.* New York, International University Press, 1963.

Dodge WT: Communication and interpersonal skills. In Taylor RB (ed): _Fundamentals of Family Medicine._ New York, Springer-Verlag, 1983.

Eble KE: _The Craft of Teaching._ San Francisco, Jossey-Bass Publishers, 1979.

Egbert LD, Battit GE, Welch CE, Bartlett MK: Reduction of postoperative pain by encouragement and instruction of patients: A study of doctor-patient rapport. _N Engl J Med_ 270: 825–827, 1964.

Eichna L: Medical school education: 1975-1979. _N Engl J Med_ 303: 727–734, 1980.

Eisner E: _The Educational Imagination._ New York, Macmillan Publishing Co., 1979.

Ellner C, Barnes CP: _Studies of College Teaching: Experimental Results, Theoretical Interpretations and New Perspectives._ Lexington, MA, D. C. Heath & Co., 1983.

Elstein AS, Shulman LS, Sprafka SA: _Medical Problem Solving._ Cambridge, MA, Harvard University Press, 1978.

Ende J: Feedback in clinical medical education. _JAMA_ 250: 777–781, 1983.

Engel GL: Clinical observation: The neglected basic method of medicine. _JAMA_ 192: 149–160, 1965.

Engel GL: Enduring attributes of medicine relevant for the education of the physician. _Ann Int Med_ 78: 587–593, 1973.

Ericksen SC, Riskind S: The interaction between teacher and student. Center for Research on Learning and Teaching (University of Michigan, Ann Arbor), Memo to the Faculty, 45: 1–6, 1971.

Esposito V, Schorow M, Siegel F: A problem-oriented precepting method. _J Fam Pract_ 3: 469–473, 1983.

Flaherty RJ: A bibliography for family practice preceptorships. _Fam Med_ 15: 73, 1983.

Foley R, Smilansky J, Yonke A: Teacher-student interaction in a medical clerkship. _J Med Educ_ 54: 622–626, 1979.

Foley R, Smilansky J: _Teaching Techniques: A Handbook for Health Professions._ New York, McGraw Hill, 1980.

Frankel BL, Rosenblum S: Teaching a biopsychosocial approach on medical attending rounds. _Gen Hosp Psychiatry_ 5: 133–140, 1983.

Gil DH, Heins M, Jones PB: Perceptions of medical school faculty members and students on clinical clerkship feedback. _J Med Educ_ 59: 856–863, 1984.

Glassman E: The teacher as leader. _New Directions for Teaching and Learning._ No. 1, 1980: 31–40.

Goodson JD, Stoeckle JD, Leaf A: Primary care training in a traditional medical residency: An ambulatory care rotation. _J Med Educ_ 55: 950–952, 1980.

Gordon T: _Parent Effectiveness Training._ New York, Peter H. Wyden, 1970.

Gordon T: _Teacher Effectiveness Training._ New York, Peter H. Wyden, 1975.

Gorlin R, Zucker HD: Physicians' reactions to patients–A key to teaching humanistic medicine. _N Engl J Med_ 308: 1059–1063, 1983.

Goroll AH, Stoeckle JD, Goldfinger SE, O'Malley T, May L, Woo B, Follayttar S, Sweet

R: Residency training in primary care internal medicine–Report of an operational program. *Ann Int Med* 83: 872–877, 1975.

Greenberg LW: Teaching primary care pediatrics to pediatric residents through an office rotation. *J Med Educ* 54: 340–342, 1979.

Grover PL, Meyerowitz SM, Hardner HH, Glaser W: An HMO-based primary care curriculum for first-year medical students. *J Med Educ* 52: 338–340, 1977.

Hansen JC, Stevic RR, Warner RW Jr: *Counseling Theory and Process.* Boston, Allyn and Bacon, 1977.

Hart L, Kurtz ME: Ambulatory care medical education: A review. *J Am Osteopath Assoc* 83: 745–749, 1984.

Herwig TH: I don't know (A Piece of My Mind). *JAMA* 256: 2348, 1986.

Holcomb JD, Garner AE: *Improving Teaching in Medical Schools (A Practical Handbook)* Springfield, IL: Charles C. Thomas Publishing, 1973.

Hurst JW: The art and science of presenting a patient's problems. *Arch Intern Med* 128: 463–465, 1971.

Ingelfinger FJ: The graying of grand rounds. *New Engl J Med* 299: 772–775, 1978.

Irby D, Rakestraw P: Evaluating clinical teaching in medicine. *J Med Educ* 56: 181–186, 1981.

Irby DM: Clinical teacher effectiveness in medicine. *J Med Educ* 53: 808–815, 1978.

Kassirer JP: Teaching clinical medicine by iterative hypothesis testing. *N Engl J Med* 309: 921–923, 1983.

Katz J. *The Silent World of Doctor and Patient.* New York: The Free Press, 1984.

Kestin J: Creativity in teaching and learning. *Am Scientist* 58: 250–257, 1970.

Klass P: Facing up to 007s: Let's talk about bad medical students, those licensed to kill. *Discover* August: 20–22, 1985.

Knopke HJ, Diekelman NL: *Approaches to Teaching in the Health Sciences.* Reading, MA: Addison-Wesley, 1978.

Knox AB: Helping teachers help adults learn. In Knox AB (ed): *Teaching Adults Effectively.* New Directions for Continuing Education, no. 6: 73–100, 1980.

Knox WJ: Obtaining a Ph.D. in psychology. *American Psychologist* 25: 1026–1032, 1970.

Lamkin B, Mygdal WK, Hitchcock M: Preceptions of the ideal clinical teacher: Views of family medicine educators. Family Practice Faculty Development Center of Texas, 4: 1–4, 1983.

Larkin J et al.: Expert and novice performance in solving physics problems. *Science* 208: 1335–1342, 1980.

Ley P, Spellman MS: Communication in an outpatient setting. *Br J Soc Clin Psychol* 4: 114–116. 1965.

Ley P, Whitworth MA, Skilbeck CE, et al.: Improving doctor-patient communications in general practice. *J Roy Coll Gen Pract* 26: 720–724, 1976.

Linfors EW, Neelon FA: The case for bedside rounds. *N Engl J Med* 303: 1230–1233, 1980.

Link K, Buchsbaum D: An agenda for residency training in ambulatory care. _J Med Educ_ 59: 494–500, 1984.

Lipkin M, Quill TE, Napodano RJ: The medical interview: A core curriculum for residencies in internal medicine. _Ann Int Med_ 100: 277–284, 1984.

Lipsitz L: Reflections of a primary-care resident–The value of community experience. _Pharos_ Summer: 23–26, 1982.

London RL, Green LA: Do family medicine residents and their teachers have common goals? _J Med Educ_ 52: 140–142, 1977.

Lowman J: Mastering the Techniques of Teaching. San Francisco: Jossey-Bass, 1984.

MacDonald PJ, Bass MJ: Characteristics of highly rated family practice preceptors. _J Med Educ_ 58: 882–893, 1983.

Machlup F: Poor learning from good teachers. _Academe:_ Oct: 376–380, 1979.

Mangold MM, Zaki EP: _Annette Garrett Interviewing: Its Principles and Methods._ New York: Family Service Association of America, 1982.

Mann RD, Arnold S, Binder J, Cytrynbaum S, Newman BM, Ringwald B, Ringwald J, Rosenwein R: _The College Classroom: Conflict, Change, and Learning._ New York, Wiley, 1970.

Margon M: Strengthening the teaching role in residency training. _J Am Med Women's Assoc_ 34: 89–91, 1979.

Mattern WD, Weinholtz D, Friedman CP: The attending physician as teacher. _N Engl J Med_ 308: 1129–1132, 1983.

McDermott W: Education and general medical care. _Ann Int Med_ 96: 512–517, 1982.

McGlynn TJ, Wynn JB, Munzenrider RF: Resident education in primary care: How residents learn. _J Med Educ_ 53: 973–981, 1978.

McKeachie WJ: _Teaching Tips._ Lexington, MA: Heath, 1965.

McLagan P: _Helping Others Learn._ Reading, MA: Addison-Wesley, 1978.

Miller GE: _Educating Medical Teachers._ Cambridge, MA: Harvard University Press, 1980.

Mouw DR: Using the personal (very personal) anecdote. _New Directions for Teaching and Learning_ 7: 27–30, 1981.

Naftulin DH, Ware JE, Donnelly FA: The Doctor Fox lecture: A paradigm of educational seduction. _J Med Educ_ 48: 630–635, 1973.

Norman D: What goes on in the mind of the learner. _New Directions for Teaching and Learning_ 2: 39, 1980.

Olness K: Teaching ambulatory pediatrics in a university HMO. _J Med Educ_ 50: 687–689, 1975.

Osborne AF: _Applied Imagination._ New York, Scribners, 1963.

Papper S: The creative clinician. _Arch Intern Med_ 144: 2049–2050, 1984.

Pawlson LG, Schroeder SA, Donaldson MS: Medical student instructional costs in a primary care clerkship. _J Med Educ_ 54: 551–555, 1979.

Payson HE, Barchas JD: A time study of medical teaching rounds. _N Engl J Med_ 273: 1468–1471, 1965.

Peitzman SJ: Lecturing in American medical schools: Tenacious tradition. *Arch Intern Med* 143: 1593–1596, 1983.

Penta FB, Kofman S: The effectiveness of emulation devices in teaching selected skills of physical diagnosis. *J Med Educ* 48: 442–445, 1973.

Perkoff GT: Teaching clinical medicine in the ambulatory setting—An idea whose time may have finally come. *N Engl J Med* 314: 27–31, 1986.

Pestana C: Sudden upper abdominal pain. In Cutler P (ed): *Problem Solving in Clinical Medicine*. Baltimore, Williams & Wilkins, 1985.

Personnel Journal: Conscious Competency–The Mark of a Competent Instructor. July 538–539, 1974.

Posner RB: Physician-patient communication. *Am J Med* 77: 59–63, 1984.

Pratt D, Magill MK: Educational contracts: A basis for effective clinical teaching. *J Med Educ* 58: 462–467, 1983.

Prial F: Accounting for tastes. *NY Times Mag* Sep 9: 103, 1984.

Proger S: A career in ambulatory medicine. *N Engl J Med* 292: 1318–1324, 1975.

Pupa LE, Carpenter JL: Morning report—A successful format. *Arch Intern Med* 145: 897–899, 1985.

Putnam SM, Wyse DH, Lawrence RS: A model for teaching primary care in a rural health center. *J Med Educ* 50: 285–287, 1975.

Raimi RA: Twice-told tale—The joy of teaching. The New York Times Spring Survey of Education. April 26, 1981, p. 59.

Reader GG, Pratt L, Mudd MC: What patients expect from their doctors. *Mod Hosp* 89: 88–94, 1957.

Reichsman F, Browning FE, Hinshaw JR: Observations of undergraduate clinical teaching in action. *J Med Educ* 39: 147–163, 1964.

Reif R: Connoisseurship in Windsor chairs. *NY Times* Mar 28: 1982.

Reuler JB, Girard DE, Nardone DA: The attending physician—Privilege and pitfalls. *JAMA* 243: 235–236, 1980.

Rogers C: *Client-Centered Therapy*. Boston, Houghton Mifflin, 1951.

Rogers DE: Some musings on medical education: Is it going astray? *Pharos* Spring, 1982.

Romano J: Patients' attitudes and behavior in ward round teaching. *JAMA* 117: 664–667, 1941.

Rowe MB: Wait time and rewards as instructional variables, their influence on language, logic, and rate control: Part 1—wait-time. *J Res Sci Teach* 11: 81–94, 1974.

Rubeck RF, Pratt DD: Conducting case-based discussions. *Ariz Med Educator* 8: 1–4, 1979.

Russell IJ et al.: Effects of three types of lecture notes on medical student achievement. *J Med Educ* 58: 627–636, 1983.

Schatz IJ: Ambulatory care training—The myth and the reality. *Arch Intern Med* 145: 1255–1256, 1985.

Schwenk TL, Detmer DE: Whither primary care in the academic medical center? *J Fam Pract:* 23: 489–493 1986.

Schwenk TL, Hughes CC: The family as the unit of care: Rhetoric or reality. *Soc Sci Med:* 17: 1–16 1983.

Schwenk TL, Whitman NA: Residents as Teachers: A Guide to Educational Practice. Salt Lake City, University of Utah School of Medicine, 1984.

Scriver M: The methodology of Evaluation. In AERA *Monograph Series on Curriculum Evaluation,* no. 1, Stake RE (ed.), Chicago: Rand McNally, 1967.

Shapiro J: A revisionist theory for the integration of behavioral science into family practice department. *J Fam Pract* 10: 275–282, 1980.

Skeff KM, Campbell M, Stratos G, Jones III H, Cooke M: Assessment by attending physicians of a seminar method to improve clinical teaching. *J Med Educ* 59: 944–950, 1984.

Skinner BF: *Walden Two.* New York, Macmillan Co., 1948.

Stein M: *Stimulating Creativity. Volume 1: Individual Procedures.* New York, Academic Press, 1974.

STFM Task Force on Behavioral Science: Behavioral science in family medicine residents: Part I, Teachers and curricula *Fam Med.* 17: 64–69, 1985.

Stillman PL, Ruggill JS, Rutala PJ, Sabers DL: Patient instructors as teachers and evaluators. *J Med Educ* 55: 186–193, 1980.

Strain JJ, Hamerman D: Ombudsmen (medical-psychiatric) rounds—An approach to meeting patient-staff needs. *Ann Int Med* 88: 550–555, 1978.

Stritter FT, Baker RM, Shahady EJ: Clinical instruction. In McGaghie WC, Frey JJ (eds): *Handbook for the Academic Physician.* New York, Springer-Verlag, 1986, pp. 98–124.

Stritter FT, Baker RM: Resident preferences for the clinical teaching of ambulatory care. *J Med Educ* 57: 33–41, 1982.

Stritter FT, Hain JD, Grimes DA: Clinical teaching reexamined. *J Med Educ* 50: 876–882, 1975.

Stritter FT, Hain, JH: A workshop in clinical teaching. *J Med Educ* 52: 155–157, 1977.

Stuart J, Rutherford RJD: Medical student concentration during lectures. *Lancet* Sept. 2: 514–516, 1978.

Tatelbaum RC, Regenstreif DI: An ambulatory training model for an obstetrics and gynecology residency program. *J Med Educ* 53: 344–351, 1978.

Tibbles L: The accuracy of supervisors' perceptions of family practice residents' educational needs. *Fam Med* 17:13–16, 1985.

Verby JE, Schaefer MT, Voeks RS: Learning forestry out of the lumberyard—A training alternative for primary care. *JAMA* 246: 645–647, 1981.

Wallas G: *The Art of Thought.* New York, Harcourt Press, 1926.

Ware J, Williams RG: The Doctor Fox effect: A study of lecturer effectiveness and ratings of instruction. *J Med Educ* 50: 149–155, 1975.

Weed LL: Medical records that guide and teach. *NEJM* 278: 593–599, 652–657, 1968.

Weiner S, Nathanson M: Physical examination: Frequently observed errors. *JAMA* 236: 852–855, 1976.

Weinholtz D: Directing medical student clinical case presentations. *Med Educ* 17: 364–368, 1983.

Whiting CS: *Creative Thinking*. New York, Reinhold Press, 1958.

Whitman NA: Choosing and using methods of teaching. Performance and Instruction 20: 16–19, 1981.

Whitman NA: *There Is No Gene for Good Teaching: A Handbook on Lecturing for Medical Teachers*. Salt Lake City, University of Utah School of Medicine, 1982.

Whitman NA, Ferrey A: "Effective medical teaching as characterized by medical school teaching award winners." Presented at the Annual Mtg. of the American Educational Research Assn. April 16, 1986, San Francisco.

Whitman NA, Schwenk TL: *A Handbook for Group Discussion Leaders: Alternatives to Lecturing Medical Students to Death*. Salt Lake City, University of Utah School of Medicine, 1983.

Whitman NA, Schwenk TL: *Preceptors as Teachers: A Guide to Clinical Teaching*. Salt Lake City, University of Utah School of Medicine, 1984.

Whitman NA, Schwenk TL: Problem solving in medical education. Can it be taught? Current Surgery November-December: 453–459, 1986.

Whitman NA, Spendlove DC, Clarke C: *Student Stress: Effects and Solutions*. Washington DC: Clearinghouse on Higher Education and Association for the Study of Higher Education, 1984.

Whitman NA: A total information learning system. Focus on Surgical Education, 2: 14–15, 1985.

Whitman NA: Teaching problem-solving and creativity in college courses. *AAHE Bull* 36: 9–13, 1983.

Williams WC: On consultation and teaching in the clinical setting. Family Practice Faculty Development Center of Texas 1: 1–4, 1980.

Wolverton, SE, Bosworth MF: A survey of resident perceptions of effective teaching behaviors. *Fam Med* 17: 106–108, 1985.

Woods D: On teaching problem solving. *Chem Eng Educ* 70: 277–284, 1979.

Wray MP, Friedland JA: Detection and correction of house staff error in physical diagnosis. *JAMA* 249: 1035–1037, 1983.

Yurchak PM: A guide to medical case presentations. *Resident Staff Physician* Sep: 109–115, 1981.

Zander AF: The discussion period in a college classroom. Memo to the Faculty, no. 62. Ann Arbor: Center for Research on Learning and Teaching, The University of Michigan, 1979.

Index

Numbers in *italics* denote figures.